Tenacity in Children

Sam Goldstein · Robert B. Brooks

Tenacity in Children

Nurturing the Seven Instincts for Lifetime Success

With a Foreword by David Crenshaw, Ph.D.

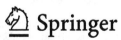 Springer

Sam Goldstein
Department of Psychiatry
University of Utah School of Medicine
Salt Lake City, UT, USA

Robert B. Brooks
Department of Psychiatry
Harvard Medical School
Needham, MA, USA

ISBN 978-3-030-65088-9   ISBN 978-3-030-65089-6   (eBook)
https://doi.org/10.1007/978-3-030-65089-6

This Springer imprint is published by the registered company Springer Nature Switzerland AG
The registered company address is: Gewerbestrasse 11, 6330 Cham, Switzerland

Say yes if your instincts are strong, even if everyone around you disagrees.

—Eve Ensler

Life is like music, it must be composed by ear, feeling and instinct, not by rule.

—Samuel Butler

In three words I can sum up everything I've learned about life: it goes on.

—Robert Frost

This book is dedicated to the children and families we have seen in assessment, consultation, and psychotherapy, and to the many talented scientists and practitioners whose ideas and work we cite in this book. You have all contributed significantly to our understanding of the seven instincts comprising Tenacity.

—Sam Goldstein and Robert B. Brooks

It's rare that one is blessed with two charismatic people in their life from whom they gather strength and learn new things; and with whom they share ideas and experience the many joys of humanity. I am fortunate to have two; my darling wife Sherrie and my dear friend and co-author Bob Brooks.

—Sam Goldstein

I dedicate this book to my wife Marilyn, my sons Rich and Doug, my daughter-in-law Suzanne, and my grandchildren Maya, Teddy, Sophie, and Lyla, whose presence and love continue to enrich my life in countless ways. And, to my dear colleague, Sam Goldstein. Little did we realize when we first met almost 30 years ago what a rich and productive journey we were destined to take.

—Robert B. Brooks

Foreword

During their remarkable, respective careers, two psychologists in particular have had and continue to exert an astonishing influence on the diverse fields of child development, clinical treatment of children, parenting, and education. Drs. Sam Goldstein and Robert B. Brooks build on their pioneering work and writings on resilience in children in their latest book, *Tenacity in Children: Nurturing the Seven Instincts for Lifetime Success*. These pioneers were among the first to identify the traits and qualities of resilient children, and how teachers, parents, and therapists can nurture and facilitate the development and strengthening of these assets. In the evolution of their work, they followed with an integration of findings regarding a fundamental building block of resilience: self-discipline whether in the context of the home, school, or psychotherapy. Once again, parents, teachers, therapists, and most of all children were the beneficiaries of their research, writings, and frequent lectures and presentations throughout the USA and internationally.

Of merit is their emphasis in recent years of the mindset of adults capable of fostering strengths and optimism in children. One of the compelling features of their research findings and writings about resilience is its transtheoretical nature; thus, a resilient mindset can be adopted by a parent, a teacher, and/or a psychotherapist regardless of any particular approach to which we adhere. A resilient mindset is adaptable to context and a wide range of settings such as home, classroom, psychotherapy office, soccer field, or dance stage. Not only is the concept of a "resilient mindset" transtheoretical, but it is also trans-contextual.

The emphasis of Goldstein and Brooks in prior writings and teachings on the identification and strengthening of *islands of competence* is a concept that holds the power to inform our work with children regardless of context. Originally introduced by Dr. Brooks as a metaphor to seek strengths in youth as a clinical strategy, such a guiding principle can inform and empower the work of all who interact with children in any substantial way. Children validate over and over the wisdom of this construct; we simply progress further by accentuating strengths in children rather than pouncing on deficits. This concept most certainly has served as a powerful force in my work.

Frequently, I sit in Treatment Planning meetings regarding children during which the vision of team members is obscured by all that is lacking in the child. The majority of their efforts are focused on defining what is "wrong" with the child rather than identifying and reinforcing what is "right." This narrow approach impedes their ability to observe the amazing talents and creativity in the child. A recent example of the robust excitement and advantage of pursuing *islands of competence* emerged in the context of an initial interview with a youth admitted to the emergency group foster care program at the agency where I serve as Clinical Director. During the interview, this 15-year-old, who I will call Jenny, shared the story of her tumultuous family life that ultimately led to her running away from home. Jenny suffered other traumatic losses and betrayals adding up to a very elevated score on the Adverse Childhood Experiences (ACEs) questionnaire and a diagnostic picture of complex interpersonal trauma. I appreciate the broad clinical expertise of the authors over careers spanning five decades as reflected in their description of working with youngsters like Jenny: "We discovered that some children demonstrated the travails of biblical Job."

Jenny's somber mood dramatically changed, however, when I inquired about her interests and talents. This chronically depressed adolescent became animated, energized, and enthused while talking about her passion for cooking. She described in exquisite detail her specialty dishes ranging from seafood to a variety of ethnic foods. I asked if she would like to cook a special dinner for her cottage. She responded with a genuine smile. She asked enthusiastically to do so as soon as possible. After walking Jenny back to her cottage, I spoke to one of the senior Youth Counselors about Jenny's avid interest in cooking and her desire to make a special dinner for her peers and staff in the group. The Youth Counselor committed to working with Jenny to go grocery shopping and obtain what was needed to cook her dinner. The next day, I delivered a stack of culinary magazines that my wife, Mary, was ready to part with to provide Jenny with material to reinforce her interests. Pursuing Jenny's *island of competence* invited her to display a side of her personhood that perhaps I would not have discovered in that initial interview and enabled us to plan interventions to support these strengths in the course of her treatment.

In this latest elaboration of their work, Goldstein and Brooks develop in meticulous detail the integrative concept of tenacity, and its underpinnings, the seven instincts. They provide a wealth of practical examples from their clinical work, including consulting and training teachers and parents. The seven instincts, defined and elaborated on in the chapters of this book, contribute the threads to the fabric that integrate tenacity into a remarkable tapestry of resilience. The holistic tapestry outlined in this book appreciates that "resilience is a process of competent functioning under duress and self-discipline is the inner control required to be resilient over time. Tenacity is the strength of will, strong mindedness, and sense of purpose needed to fuel self-discipline and resilience."

Many researchers have helped to illuminate the nature of resilience starting with Robert White, Michael Rutter, Norman Garmezy, Emmy Werner, Suniya Luthar, Ann Masten, Michael Ungar, and many other seminal thinkers. Without diminishing the important contributions of those listed and others, the astonishing gift of Drs. Goldstein and Brooks is their ability to translate the theory and research from the resilience field into language, friendly to a wide range of practitioners in mental health and child development disciplines as well as parents and educators. This broad reach and the ability to offer practical strategies that can be employed in a wide range of contexts by parents and child helpers of many disciplines, and different levels of training make their work of extraordinary impact. Yet another incredibly helpful aspect of their work is the identification of obstacles that frequently emerge in the path to achieving the goals set and useful ways to cope with such potential roadblocks. This component can be particularly supportive of the efforts of dedicated parents and teachers who may be doing all the right things but the changes they work toward in the child may take longer and require more patience than they originally anticipated.

Perhaps the most important characteristic of Drs. Goldstein and Brooks' cumulative writings on resilience is their highly sensitive and respectful approach to parents and teachers. These dedicated adults invest heart and soul into their efforts to guide children yet are not always successful. The contributing factors to child development are multi-determined, complex, and sometimes beyond our understanding. Too often, parents, teachers, and sometimes psychotherapists are blamed when treatment does not progress as desired. In many instances, the path forward is complex, not well understood, nor readily apparent. This book is a rich contribution to a more complete understanding of the complicated process by which children become who they are and the means to find that path.

By way of a brief preview, I want to comment on the instinct of Intuitive Optimism introduced in Chapter 3. The authors recommend a practical strategy: engaging children in contributory activities. They support this recommendation in part based on their research about what people report as their happiest memories from their school experiences. While the findings may surprise some readers, those who adopt a resilient mindset will find it validating that most often people in the survey mentioned experiences of helping out in some way even if it were something so simple as taking the attendance list to the office at school. Helping in some way enables children to feel they are contributing and that they have something to offer to others, which then reinforces their sense of belonging. This is one of the features of Drs. Goldstein and Brooks' decades of work on resilience that I value the most because you don't need to apply for a $100,000 grant, hire more staff, or obtain more training or equipment to ask children to help out in some way to elevate their spirit.

I want to provide two more examples from my clinical experiences of the groundbreaking impact of the work of these distinguished scholars and authors. My agency, the Children's Home of Poughkeepsie, invited Dr. Brooks to be our featured speaker in 2015 when we organized a conference about "Resilience in Children." As mentioned previously, these authors in addition to their demanding clinical work and writing offer numerous presentations and trainings on many aspects of resilience both nationally and internationally. Dr. Brooks in his usual charismatic way enthralled the audience with his eloquent presentation on resilience laced with humor and riveting stories. As a result of the foundation laid by the education, training, and writings of these two remarkable psychologists, I was able to require, with little resistance, that all of the treatment plans at our agency contain a new section titled "Islands of Competence." The initial treatment plan is updated each quarter including any additions of strengths, interests, and talents we have recently discovered in the young person.

A second modification to our program based on inspiration from Drs. Goldstein and Brooks was to our Sanctuary Model, a trauma-informed organizational approach created by Sandra Bloom, M.D. Integral to the Sanctuary Model are red flag meetings. Red flag meetings can be called by anyone working with a child or adolescent or the youth him or herself when there are setbacks or repeated crises suggestive of something going awry in the youth's treatment. After discussing an idea with Dr. Bloom and with her blessing, I was able to introduce green flag meetings. Green flag meetings can be called by anyone on the team or the youth to call attention to progress that a youth is making, particularly in overcoming some significant challenges or obstacles. It is an opportunity to celebrate their growth and progress and highlight their strength and determination as well as credit those who have supported the youth through a difficult time.

I fully expect that you will find this book enjoyable and rewarding. The authors make a compelling case for resilience, self-discipline, and tenacity as the essential triad of human development. As with their previous work, Drs. Goldstein and Brooks lay out the science informing their constructs, in addition to their signature practice of outlining useful interventions with clear directives to do so, illustrated by examples from their clinical practices. They effectively engage children and all who strive to work with them by replacing the medical model (pathology focused) with the resilience model (strengths focused). The former model leaves in its wake disempowered and too often defeated and hopeless youth as well as the well-meaning parents, educators and professionals who strive to help them. The resilience model championed tirelessly by these pioneering authors has injected revitalizing energy, fresh air, and empowerment into the work of helping children heal and grow in healthy ways. Books are intended to be read. In this instance reread, so I will not spoil the introduction of these new concepts and ways of thinking by writing much more except to note: This will be an extraordinary exploration into reframing your thoughts about children and who we are as a species, as you dive into the pages ahead.

Poughkeepsie, NY, USA   David A. Crenshaw, Ph.D., ABPP

Preface

Who We Are

Thousands of years ago, our Homo sapiens ancestors lived by hunting, fishing, and gathering. They took what they needed from the world around them. As nomads, they created homes in natural shelters or primitive huts. On a warm summer night 15,000 years ago, a mother and father watched as their three children frolicked alongside a small stream in a wooded landscape. They couldn't help but notice how different their three children were. The youngest, brash and bold, often found new ways to find food. The middle child, quiet, even shy, but always ready to help and make sure everyone had something to eat. Finally, the eldest was increasingly taking responsibility for the safety of the family group when the men were away hunting.

Over thousands and thousands of generations, parents prepared their children for adult life. Children learned by example. Evolution or the process of natural selection determined better adaptation and served as the foundation of parenting. Though parents taught by example not every child was an equally successful student. As with any species, this foundation evolved into a set of instincts present, but unevenly distributed, in every member of the species. These instincts enhanced survival. As species evolved so too did the complexity and importance of these instincts. In concert with the environment, these instincts became dependent upon experience to flourish and exert a positive influence on behavior.

As Matt Ridley wrote in his 2011 book *The Rational Optimist*: "At some point, human intelligence became collective and cumulative in a way that happened to no other animal." Over tens of thousands of years, this has provided us with untold advantages but at least one unexpected downside. We have failed to sufficiently appreciate the power of many human instincts in shaping child development and adult life. Whether we realized it or not, we have until recently parented and educated from the position that children are tabula rasa or blank slates waiting to be infused with knowledge.

In this book, we propose that the lengthy transition from childhood to adulthood must be built on a foundation of the seven instincts we have placed under the umbrella of *Tenacity*. We must reframe how we parent, educate, and socialize our children if we are to prepare them for a future few if any of us can imagine.

We are fortunate for our friendship over the past 30 years. As many of our peers retire or begin to limit their professional and academic work, we find ourselves at a unique and exciting time in our lives, a time during which our ideas and theories continue to evolve.

Many people have made significant contributions to our joint work. We want to thank our literary agent of nearly 25 years, James Levine, our first Editor, Matthew Carnicelli, and our current Editor at Springer, Judy Jones. All three of these individuals have appreciated and trusted our vision. We have also had the opportunity to work with many fine editors at multiple publishers shepherding our eight trade books, five textbooks, and a parenting program. Throughout all of our books as well as film, radio, research, and article projects, we have been blessed by the diligence and work of our Editorial Assistant Kathy Gardner and for this book Moana Erickson.

We are also indebted to our families, friends, and colleagues for indulging our passion to create new ideas and for never hesitating to tell us what they think about those ideas. We thank Dr. Crenshaw for his thoughtful Foreword. Finally absent the thousands of children and families seeking our help and trusting our guidance, *Tenacity in Children* would never have been written.

The many families you will meet in this book are representative of the populations with whom we have worked in our clinical practices. Though some stories are compilations of experiences, all of the examples reflect the course of events for real children and families. As such, we offer many of these stories as "we" and "our" rather than Bob or Sam.

One final point. We have written this book during one of the most challenging times in our lives and the lives of our children as reflected in the pandemic of 2020, the growing political schism in America and throughout the world and our renewed confrontation of racism. While the principles and strategies we advance are applicable at any time, they take on even greater importance as we help our children to confront these unprecedented events with increased optimism, compassion, resilience, and tenacity.

Let us remember as Neil Postman has written, "Children are the living messages we send to a time we will not see." It is our hope that the ideas, principles and strategies in this book will make a positive difference in your lives and the lives of your children today and long into the future.

Salt Lake City, USA   Sam Goldstein, Ph.D.
Needham, USA   Robert B. Brooks, Ph.D.

Praise for *Tenacity in Children*

"In *Tenacity in Children: Nurturing the Seven Instincts for Lifetime Success*, Drs. Goldstein and Brooks offer compelling evidence for a contrasting model that states that children are instinctively empathetic and motivated and the goal of caregivers is to nurture, foster, and develop these attributes in the children they serve. The collaboration of these two esteemed psychologists has been impacting on our field for decades and this new book continues that tradition."

—Richard D. Lavoie, M.A., M.Ed., Author, *It's So Much Work to Be Your Friend: Helping Children with Learning Disabilities Find Social Success*

"Drs. Goldstein and Brooks are embodiments of tenacity and its seven instincts. We see this in their clinical stories, and how they have worked over decades to use Intuitive Optimism, Intrinsic Motivation, Compassionate Empathy, Genuine Altruism, Virtuous Responsibility, and the other instincts to turn children and adolescents' islands of competence into lives of meaningful connection. The seven instincts that contribute to Tenacity can be likened to the dimensions of Multiple Intelligences and I anticipate that Tenacity will prove to be as revolutionary a concept in education and psychotherapy as MI has been. You could not ask for a more complete guide to an uplifting parenting, clinical, and educational approach that deeply respects the strength and dignity of children."

—Maurice J. Elias, Ph.D., Director, the Social-Emotional and Character Development Lab, Rutgers University; Co-author *Nurturing Students' Character: Everyday Teaching Activities for Social-Emotional Learning*

"There's a 'trick' to the book *Tenacity for Children* by Drs. Goldstein and Brooks. You might pick it up to read and absorb because you want to teach your children the seven instincts. But if you're honest, you'll also start trying to practice these for yourself as well. It's a fast read the first time through. For your second pass, bring a notebook."

—Chris Brogan, Business Advisor; Co-author, *Trust Agents*

"I took great joy learning from Goldstein and Brooks' newest book. Their evidence-based wealth of information resonated soundly with me—not only to apply to the many children I work with, but also my mature adult clients. Whether a child is 10 years old or in their 60s or 70s, they are never too old to be nurtured in their development of tenacity. And we, as parents, teachers, or counselors will be grateful, as this book shines a light on so many different ways, we the nurturers can nurture."

—Michelle Garcia Winner, MA-CCC, Founder, Social Thinking Methodology;
Author, *Thinking About You Thinking About Me*

"*Tenacity in Children* has allowed me to look at many of my experiences with children and understand the importance of approaching every challenge with a positive view of what we do well and not just what it is missing. *Tenacity in Children* is so easy to read and understand how to nurture the seven instincts to support each child's growth and of every person for that matter. *Tenacity in Children* is the perfect balance between concepts, knowledge, scientific discourse, practical ideas, and heartwarming stories that truly illustrate the principles shared in the book."

—Encarni Gallardo, MBA, CPM, Executive Director, Children's Service Society of
Utah

"In *Tenacity in Children*, Sam Goldstein and Robert Brooks make critical ideas accessible in a conversational, clinically rich, warm, and encouraging way. Understanding Intuitive Optimism, Islands of Competence, and Intrinsic Motivation helps guide us to be self-compassionate, nurture joy and persistence, and help children to develop to their full potential. They are not giving a formula or recipe but give innovative suggestions, supportive reflection, and encouragement to dialogue, reinforce a sense of personal control, and teach problem-solving strategies."

—Nancy Rappaport, M.D., Associate Professor of Psychiatry, Harvard Medical
School; Co-author, *The Behavior Code: A Practical Guide to Understanding and
Teaching the Most Challenging Students*

"Heartful and overflowing with wisdom, this practical and caring book reveals how parents can nurture their children's innate well-being and potential. Two of the kindest and most respected people in the field once again provide us with a fresh perspective on raising happy, resilient, and also tenacious kids."

—Mark Bertin, M.D., Author, *How Children Thrive*

"Written in an easy-to-read, narrative style, Drs. Goldstein and Brooks impart their innovative concept of Tenacity in Children along with its seven essential instincts by using heart-warming stories, personal and professional insights, research, and wisdom. At a time when life challenges are ever present, this book will inspire hope, provide guidance, and emphasize the need for compassion in our quest to raise resilient children and nurture our human spirit."

—Joyce C. Mills, Ph.D., Founder, StoryPlay® Global; Co-author, *Therapeutic
Metaphors for Children and the Child Within*

"The authors are leaders in this work and have crafted a much needed guide based on over 30 years of research, practice, and reflection as to what truly drives and fosters tenacity in children and how families, educators, and medical professionals can support its development."

—Katherine Dockweiller, Ed.D., Co-founder Healthy Minds, Healthy Schools Las Vegas, Nevada

"For decades, Drs. Goldstein and Brooks have made significant contributions to the field of child development. This book is no exception. However, its implications extend far beyond the clinical and educational environment, making it a valuable resource for personal and professional development. The questions posed offer a roadmap for personal reflection and for fostering tenacity in others and ourselves. In their decision to first discover the strengths of children, they provide a powerful shift in perspective. Rather than focusing on deficits, they seek to identify each child's 'island of competence.' This profound act restores the critical component of personal control—something we all need for personal transformation. This book demonstrates the power of strengths to nurture the attributes of resilience and tenacity. Whether you are a parent, a teacher, a co-worker, or a leader, this critical work matters now more than ever."

—Rob Hatch, Executive Coach; Author, *ATTENTION!*

"This book combines scientific studies, philosophical thought, and practical experience with innovative concepts and practice. As such, this book is important and significant reading material for professionals, parents and the public at large."

—Iris Manor, M.D., Associate professor, Sackler School of Medicine, Tel Aviv University, Israel

"Drs. Goldstein and Brooks connect the science behind principles that we all have experienced in an engaging way that gives us a roadmap for empowering our children to be the best they can be."

—Alan Fine, Founder, President of InsideOut Development

Contents

About the Authors

Sam Goldstein obtained his Ph.D. in School Psychology from the University of Utah and is licensed as Psychologist and certified School Psychologist in the state of Utah. He is also board certified as Pediatric Neuropsychologist and listed in the Council for the National Register of Health Service Providers in Psychology. He is Fellow of the American Psychological Association and the National Academy of Neuropsychology. He is an Adjunct Assistant Professor in the Department of Psychiatry, the University of Utah School of Medicine. He has authored, co-edited, or co-authored over fifty clinical and trade publications, three dozen chapters, nearly three dozen peer-reviewed scientific articles, and eight psychological and neuropsychological tests. Since 1980, he has served as Clinical Director of The Neurology, Learning and Behavior Center in Salt Lake City, Utah.

Robert B. Brooks obtained his Ph.D. in Clinical Psychology from Clark University in Worcester, MA, and completed a postdoctoral fellowship at the University of Colorado Medical School in Denver. He is board certified in Clinical Psychology and listed in the Council for the National Register of Health Service Providers in Psychology. He is currently on the faculty of Harvard Medical School (part-time) and is Former Director of the Department of Psychology at McLean Hospital, a private psychiatric hospital. He has authored, co-edited, or co-authored 18 books and, in addition, authored or co-authored almost three dozen chapters and more than three dozen peer-reviewed scientific articles. He has received numerous awards for his work, including most recently the Mental Health Humanitarian Award from William James College in Massachusetts for his contributions as a Clinician, Educator, and Author.

Also By These Authors:

Raising Resilient Children (2001)
Seven Steps to Help Your Child Worry Less (with Kristy Hagar) (2002)
Parenting Resilient Children Parent Training Manual (2002)
Nurturing Resilience in Our Children (2003)
The Power of Resilience (2004)
Angry Children, Worried Parents (with Sharon Weiss) (2004)
Handbook of Resilience in Children (2005)
Seven Steps to Improve Your Child's Social Skills (with Kristy Hagar) (2006)
Understanding and Managing Children's Classroom Behavior—2nd Edition (2007)
Raising a Self-Disciplined Child (2009)
Raising Resilient Children with Autism Spectrum Disorders (2012)
Handbook of Resilience in Children—2nd Edition (2012)
Play Therapy Interventions to Enhance Resilience (with David Crenshaw) (2015)
Handbook of Resilience in Children—3rd Edition (in Progress)

Chapter 1
Our Thirty-Year Journey

From a very young age, Andrew demonstrated strong symptoms of Autism Spectrum Disorder. He was socially aloof, seemed preoccupied with objects, and spent the majority of time disengaged from others. Andrew lacked the instinctual connection young children share with adults. He struggled to take the perspective of others, appeared to lack empathy, and was easily distressed.

Though Andrew slowly acquired basic social skills, he continued to demonstrate an interest in "spooning." He had a favorite wooden cooking spoon with a hole in the center that he would hold like a baton. He would wave it back and forth while periodically gazing through the hole at the world around him. While engaging in this behavior, he would move around at times in seemingly purposeless circles. Sometimes, he would chant or sing to himself. The words, however, were never discernible. If left alone he would participate in this behavior for hours on end. He didn't cry when his parents took the spoon away. Instead, he would simply substitute some other elongated object. Andrew's grandparents, absent any education about Autism, thought the behavior somehow must be important to Andrew and would bring him wooden spoons, much to the unhappiness of his parents.

We didn't understand the purpose of this behavior. Andrew, despite developing spoken language and seemingly normal intelligence by age five, was unable to provide us with any kind of explanation about the occurrence of "spooning." Andrew's parents were concerned that he would engage in this behavior at school so approximately six months before school began we used this behavior as a reinforcer. That is, Andrew could have his wooden spoon if he engaged in certain behaviors appropriately such as playing a game with his parents or sitting through dinner.

Andrew agreed not to take the spoon to school. In exchange, when he came home he was given a half hour of "spooning time." Interestingly, at school Andrew did not substitute any other object and in fact his teacher never observed him engaging in spooning behavior, even though during recess he tended to wander independently on the playground sometimes talking to himself. Andrew's use of the spoon at home decreased in the following year.

© Springer Nature Switzerland AG 2021
S. Goldstein and R. B. Brooks, *Tenacity in Children*,
https://doi.org/10.1007/978-3-030-65089-6_1

At six and a half years of age during a visit with us, he brought in a gift-wrapped package. It was the spoon. He told us he didn't "need" it any longer and we could give it to someone else who might need it. This wouldn't be the last time we visited with Andrew. In fact, Andrew returned seeking our help thirty-five years later. We will discuss Andrew's visit in Chapter 10.

A Friendship Begins

C. S. Lewis wrote: "Friendship is born at that moment when one person says to another, 'What! You too? I thought I was the only one.'" We met at a psychology conference in 1992. Over lunch, we discovered that after fifteen years of working with children and families we had arrived at a shared conclusion—we were falling far short of providing the hope and help we envisioned.

During that lunch, a rich friendship and collaboration was born. We spent hours sharing thoughts about the framework and shortcomings of our training as psychologists and an alternative, strength-based approach and perspective that we had begun to embrace. This new perspective we believed would be much more effective in improving the lives of children and adults than the one we were taught and had diligently practiced in our work. Little did we know that our endeavor to articulate this new framework would result in co-authoring or co-editing 14 science and trade books, a parenting program, countless articles, chapters, a radio series, and an award-winning documentary created for the lay public and professional audiences. In each project, we had opportunities to elaborate upon applying our ideas in our clinical work and beyond.

Our evolving perspective is in keeping with similar changes transpiring within psychology and mental health over the past 30 years as evidenced by the emergence of what has been referred to as the field of *positive psychology*. Many of the titles and content of books and articles published in clinical psychology since 1992 reflect a shift in focus that continues to take place. We have been fortunate that our ideas have resonated with so many parents and professionals. Between us, we have had the opportunity to share our ideas with countless others in all walks of life and train tens of thousands of professionals on four continents.

Tenacity in Children is an outgrowth of our continued elaboration of a strength-based model to understand human behavior and empower youth and adults. The concept of tenacity is rooted in our earlier works examining the components of resilience and self-discipline. After writing the trade books *Raising Resilient Children*, *The Power of Resilience*, and *Nurturing Resilience in Our Children*, as well as co-editing a science volume, *Handbook of Resilience in Children*, in which we introduced and elaborated on the concept of a *resilient mindset*, we recognized that one component of that mindset, self-discipline, deserved separate attention. This prompted us to further research and author *Raising a Self-Disciplined Child*.

We appreciate that resilience is a process of competent functioning under duress and self-discipline is the inner control required to be resilient over time. In our continued work with children and families, we recognized that the guideposts of resilience and self-discipline were always helpful but at times fell short of our goals. Through our professional and personal experience, we learned that functional behavior and self-control over time require a certain kind of determination and a firm grip in charting life decisions. This is what tenacity represents. Tenacity is the strength of will, strong mindedness, and sense of purpose needed to fuel self-discipline and resilience. Tenacity is rooted in a mindset of stalwart belief.

Our goal in writing this book is to introduce the concept of tenacity and define the ways in which it is interwoven with and an elaboration of the earlier concepts we have addressed. In this book, we continue our journey of thirty years. We will address the third of what we consider the *essential triad of human development*—resilience, self-discipline, and tenacity. To help you fully understand the shifts in our thinking during the past several decades, we think it will be helpful to briefly describe the research and experiences that encouraged us to alter our path multiple times during our professional journey.

The Medical Model

In our work in tertiary care programs (those for children with very serious problems), we discovered that some children demonstrated the travails of biblical Job. These children did not just face one or two adversities but multiple challenges, each of which alone caused impairment in many areas of life, but together resulted in significant disruption in school, on the playground, and within the family. We were trained by our supervisors in the *medical model*. The very same model in which they were trained. Simply put, this model focuses on identifying and fixing what is wrong in people. For these children, our quest to find and fix their problems was overwhelming.

The primary premise of a *medical model* approach seems at first glance to be admirable, namely if you fix what is wrong in people you even the playing field of life for them. Little did we appreciate that such a premise created blinders, constricting our view of the whole person. We possessed 20–20 vision in our search for pathology, but we spent little, if any, time seeking the strengths that resided in each individual. As mental health professionals we were very well trained in finding problems within the children and adults with whom we worked. In fact, we were so well trained that we could find at least something wrong with everyone!

It is understandable that the *medical model* was adapted to mental health care. After all, mental health care has typically been an extension of medical care, particularly since the first mental health professionals were in fact physicians. Psychiatry is an entire field developed from physical medicine, focused specifically on mental health. But today, the majority of mental health professionals are not physicians. In fact, many psychiatrists, while providing medical care by prescribing psychiatric medications, do not engage in other forms of mental health care.

During our careers, we have come to realize assessing what is wrong with you may yield information about your current life and the challenges you face; however, what is right about you in a variety of domains—general development, interests, emotions, behavior, intellect, relations to others, to name but a few—tells us much more about what you may and can accomplish in life. We have steadily shifted away from a medical model seeking to know what is wrong and fixing it, to a comprehensive, holistic model appreciating that symptom relief is necessary to relieve immediate problems and impairment but is insufficient to help challenged children transition happily and successfully into their adult lives. This idea formed the foundation for our first book, *Raising Resilient Children*. This is an outcome all parents hope and wish for their children.

A Shift to a Resilience Model

We replaced the *medical model* with a *resilience model*. We have developed an appreciation that learning to cope is but the first step in continuing to function well in the presence of any adversity and, more importantly, to successfully transition into adult life. We have come to understand that biology is not destiny, despite the fact that it affects probability. We are aware that our genes determine the borders of the playing field of our lives. But we also recognize that our experiences shape how and in what manner these genes express themselves and ultimately where our lives take us in what turns out to be a vast field of possibilities.

In our work, we have had the opportunity to watch the first children with whom we worked grow up and raise children of their own. In fact, we have seen the grandchildren of some of our first cases! We have been honored that these families have chosen to bring their children and grandchildren to see us. We have not been surprised by their struggles since many of the conditions we have treated have a strong genetic basis, increasing the likelihood that future generations will require assistance.

The Shortcomings of Prediction

Our ability to predict adult outcome was not as accurate as we initially believed. Some of the children we evaluated and worked with, whose parents were understandably worried about their future given the struggles they faced in their childhood, were doing very well as adults. Others who seemed on a more positive trajectory during their child and adolescent years, in part because of the significant support they received, were struggling in adulthood, unable to find a comparable level of support and care.

Similar accounts can be seen in the journeys of children who were never under a therapist's care, such as those who struggled as youngsters but were doing well as adults or those whose benign childhood stories would not have foreseen the emotional burdens they faced in adulthood. And, of course, there were those whose adult lives, whether positive or negative, were an extension of their earlier years.

The question we faced as mental health professionals was how to understand these trajectories and, when needed, alter these different paths in life for the better. We learned that parents came to see us not only because they were worried about their children's current challenges but even more so about how an adverse present may affect the future. Parents were eager for us to gaze into the eyes of their children, make predictions about the future, and if those predictions were dire, to set out today to change the future.

We now know, as noted above, that fixing what is wrong, while necessary to relieve symptoms, does not in and of itself exert a significant positive influence in changing the future. For example, children with Attention Deficit Hyperactivity Disorder (ADHD) taking medicine throughout their childhood do not appear to transition into adulthood with significantly fewer risks or adversities than children with ADHD who never took medication. It is not that the medicine is unhelpful, but that the medicine alone is insufficient to accomplish parents' goals in seeking our help, simply put, to help their children transition happily and successfully into adult life.

How the Brain and Mind Work

Among our most challenging therapeutic tasks has been to explain to parents, education and medical professionals, even children, how the brain and mind work. In the past, for example, when a child struggled to learn to read we told parents their child suffered from a reading disorder. When parents asked what led to this conclusion, we were left to offer a rather simplistic response, "Because they are struggling to read." Fortunately, during the past forty years, the science of neuropsychology has begun to provide more sophisticated answers to this and other developmental challenges children face. With this knowledge, effective teaching and therapy strategies are being developed.

After thousands of evaluations, we have come to understand and appreciate the differences between the developing brain and the mind, as well the difference between ability, knowledge, and skill. In fact, when parents bring their children to us to conduct an initial evaluation, these differences are one of the first things we discuss with them and set out to evaluate. Diagnoses, though valuable, are no longer a sufficient explanation for the many problems children may experience. The goal of our assessment is not to add up symptoms and proclaim diagnoses, but rather to assist parents, educators, physicians, and other adults in children's lives to see the world through the eyes of the child. To do this, we help them understand that our initial view of the child's developing brain focuses on three phenomena:

Ability: Abilities are the genetically driven, biological qualities all of us bring to the world. These qualities are not evenly distributed among people. That is, some of us are better and some of us are weaker in many of these qualities. These qualities include not only physical abilities (e.g., balance and coordination) but also cognitive abilities (memory, reasoning, thinking, attention, planning, sequencing, etc.). Abilities are in fact hardwired. This does not mean we cannot assist children with weaker abilities to strengthen these abilities and be successful in life; rather, we recognize that although some children may not attain proficiency in certain abilities, all children can be successful if we are sufficiently enlightened. We also recognize that it is equally important to identify and build on those abilities that represent their strengths.

Knowledge: Knowledge is all that you learn by experience. It is much more than just academics. For example, language is knowledge. If you do not speak to children, they will never speak. Socialization is dependent on knowledge. A child may have all the genetics needed to socialize appropriately but if never given the opportunity to interact with other children will not know how to do so. Our abilities help us acquire knowledge. For some children, this may be an accelerated process while for others as Dr. Joan Goodman has written, *slow is fast enough.* We have learned how to help parents change their minds and adjust their expectations for the pace at which their child will acquire knowledge, emotional regulation, and self-discipline and even socialize.

Skill: We use our abilities to acquire knowledge. However, possessing knowledge and ability is just the foundation. We must skillfully apply these two to solve problems in all walks of life. In our perspective, skill is not a noun (e.g., reading skill) but a verb (e.g., skillfully reading). All kinds of factors can impair skill. Some children may possess excellent coordination and be very good athletes but not skillful in competition because they are nervous, impulsive, or ill-prepared. Other children may possess average ability to sequence and associate and are average readers but are very successful at school because they are skillful in meeting all of their school responsibilities.

An appreciation of these developmental phenomena—ability, knowledge, and skill—provides a firm, reasoned, and reasonable means of understanding our children as well as ourselves. If you are uncertain of your children's ability, knowledge, and skill, a comprehensive neuropsychological evaluation can help to better understand the source of problems as well as strengths, and guide remedial and compensatory support.

Gifts from Our Children

We have often heard mental health professionals (and teachers) express the view that they have learned more from their patients (and students) than the latter have learned from them. As we reflect upon the many children, parents, and other adults we have seen for evaluation and psychotherapy from the time we were first in training, we are well aware of how much we learned from them. In our collaboration, we have laughed about children and families who seemed to be sent our way to convey the following message: "The medical model you're using is shortsighted. It's keeping you from being an effective psychotherapist. Let me guide you to adopt a strength-based approach that will bring greater satisfaction and success in your work and will be much more beneficial to me and other patients."

To appreciate the "gifts" we've received from our work and the ways in which these gifts served as catalysts guiding us along new paths from a medical to a resilience model, we want to share several stories from our clinical work. Each story exemplifies how misguided we were in our efforts to help and the important lessons we learned.

Baseball is more interesting than math. Adam was the very first child Sam was asked to administer an intelligence test to during his postgraduate training. Sam was informed that Adam was difficult to evaluate. It was Sam's job to administer the intelligence test over the coming hour. Sam had no idea what to expect other than the child's mother described her son as hyperactive, impulsive, and inattentive. Sure enough, as Sam attempted to begin administering the intelligence test, Adam had a difficult time remaining seated. He frequently looked around the room, stood up, made unrelated comments, and did not appear to be listening as Sam read the task instructions.

Sam repeatedly redirected Adam to the test, but Adam would only focus for short periods of time. At one point, Adam took a stack of baseball cards out of his pocket and put them on the table.

He asked Sam, "Do you like baseball?"

In a moment of creativity or maybe desperation, Sam abandoned the test and instead began asking Adam questions about the baseball cards. Suddenly, Adam sat still, paid attention to the conversation, and stayed on task. He proceeded to show the baseball cards to Sam, explaining the differences in players' positions, batting averages, and teams.

During the next 15 minutes, Adam was completely engrossed in discussing his baseball cards with Sam. Sam quickly realized that Adam's problem was not so much that he could not pay attention, sit still, or control his impulses, but that he required a much higher level of interest and motivation to bring these qualities "online." As Sam attempted to return to the intelligence test, Adam quickly regressed to his previous level of behavior.

Adam's behavior was an important initial lesson for Sam. Many of the behavioral problems we describe in children are not in fact set in stone nor evident in all situations. Rather, these behaviors are very influenced by what is taking place around the child as well as the child's interests and mindset.

Sam's insight was not appreciated by his Supervisor. He was admonished for allowing Adam to dictate the testing session and for not completing the intelligence test due to Adam's inattention. Having worked with rats before he decided he liked children better, Sam attempted to explain to his Supervisor that perhaps like some of his rats, Adam could pay attention when the task was sufficiently engaging, of interest to him, or had a valued payoff. He simply required a higher level of interest to engage. Sam suggested our field needed more interesting tests for children like Adam. Sam was informed that he was wrong. Years later, researchers would demonstrate that even the most inattentive child will pay attention with the right mindset, under the right environmental circumstances.

"We're going to outlast you!" One of the most challenging positions Bob ever held took place at the beginning of his career. He was appointed Principal of a school in the locked door unit of a child and adolescent program in a psychiatric hospital. He often questions whether he had sufficient experience to assume such a demanding post, but he appreciates that what he learned from these students provided him with an invaluable, sometimes painful, education.

Unprepared for the intense acting-out behaviors of a number of these youth, Bob and his staff adopted a reactive mode; that is, they mainly focused on what to do when outbursts occurred rather than asking, "What might we do to lessen the emergence of these behaviors?" In addition, this reactive mentality led to forms of discipline that were rooted in the belief, "I'll show you who's in charge here!" Bob was to learn that when staff felt they were losing control, they often resorted to becoming more controlling via an increased number of rules and harsher consequences.

Seth was a 12-year-old boy admitted to the hospital for his physical outbursts and aggression. Not surprisingly, he continued these behaviors at the hospital. On seven consecutive school days, Bob placed him in the "quiet" or "time-out" room in response to an outburst. Seth's behavior did not change, nor did Bob's.

On the eighth day, Seth angrily asked, "Why do you keep putting me in the quiet room?"

Not knowing what to say, Bob offered an intellectual response, something to the effect of, "The quiet room is a place for you to reflect on your behaviors so you can change them."

Seth cursed and then shouted, "You don't get it, do you Brooks!"

"Get what?" Bob asked.

"We're going to outlast you!"

This and similar comments from several other students at the school were turning points in Bob's recognition that he really "didn't get it," that, for example, what he called discipline focused exclusively on punishment rather than teaching, that his approach was based on finding ways of "controlling" children, rather than reinforcing self-discipline. Not only had he not realized this but he had also failed to identify and employ their interests and strengths. In the following months, Bob and the rest of the staff were to make changes in this approach, resulting in a positive change in the behavior of the students. Rather than dictating the rules unilaterally, youth in the program were asked to offer their ideas about rules and the consequences for breaking them. Though not all recommendations were adopted, Bob was surprised at the level of responsibility these youth displayed when given the opportunity to be heard. Bob's favorite memory was starting a "Space Committee" tasked with making sure furnishings and other materials were properly treated at the recommendation of a youth prone to destructive behavior when angry. This boy suggested he be placed on this Committee because he knew "all the ways to break things!"

"You came to my game!" Cynthia, a 14-year-old girl, was referred to Bob by her middle school counselor. The counselor described her as "very bright and athletic, but also prone to physical outbursts when angered by another student." The event that led to the referral occurred when Cynthia and another girl became involved in a shoving match. The other girl fell backward and was briefly dazed when she struck her head against the wall. She was revived quickly. Fortunately, there were no obvious adverse effects.

During the first few months of therapy with Bob, Cynthia constantly complained that she didn't want to see him, and the only reason she came was that her school counselor told her that if she wanted to remain on the soccer team—her favorite sport and a sport at which she excelled—she needed to be in therapy (the counselor told Bob that he had told Cynthia that she needed to be in therapy to learn to handle her outbursts, but had not made it a condition of her playing soccer). In her sessions with Bob, Cynthia would often blame others for her outbursts. Alternately, she would remain silent for long periods of time.

Yet, she continued to see Bob, perhaps knowing that she needed help managing her anger. While Cynthia had spoken some about her love of soccer, during one meeting she surprised Bob by asking, "Why don't you ever come to one of my soccer games?"

Bob wondered, "Why would you want me to come?"

Cynthia said, "You'd see what a good player I am."

This led to a lengthy discussion of Cynthia's strengths and whether Bob and others were aware of some of these strengths.

Cynthia asked again, "Can you come to one of my games? I have one this Saturday morning. You don't even have to come for the entire game."

It was obvious how much Bob attending even part of her soccer game meant to Cynthia. Bob knew it wouldn't require much of his time since he and Cynthia lived in the same town and the soccer field was only a mile away. What was more of an issue for Bob was hearing the admonitions of his former supervisors' saying, "You should never see a patient outside the office or share personal information, it might interfere with the progress of therapy."

Bob understood that he had to be cautious when having an interaction with a child outside the office, but in considering Cynthia's request, he sensed how important it was for her to have him observe her engaged in a favored activity; he also knew that given all of the adults attending the game, he could remain anonymous on the sidelines.

Bob attended the game and what transpired was the kind of event of which Hollywood movies are made. At one point, an opposing player tripped Cynthia. Cynthia got up and approached the girl. Bob thought, "Oh no, she's going to hit that girl!" Instead, Cynthia in a relatively calm voice said to this girl, "You're going to pay for tripping me!" With little time left in the game, Cynthia dribbled past the girl, scored the winning goal, and said to her, "I told you that you were going to pay."

At the next session, Cynthia told Bob, "I'm glad you came." Bob replied that he was glad he could be there, that he was very impressed with Cynthia's soccer skills, but there was an incident that transpired about which he was even more impressed.

Cynthia wondered, "What's that?"

Bob noted that when the girl tripped her and she went up to the girl, he was very impressed that she kept her cool and didn't try to push the girl.

Cynthia interrupted and with a smile said, "Dr. Brooks, I would never do that. If I retaliated I could be kicked out of the game."

Although this conversation was replete with humor, its content touched upon a very serious subject, namely Cynthia's mindset and the factors that triggered her anger as well as what she might do to control her emotions in different situations beyond the soccer field.

Bob recognized that attending Cynthia's soccer game and witnessing her strengths or what he was to call her "islands of competence" was a catalyst to form a therapeutic alliance that was to yield very positive results. Little did Bob know how significant an event it was. We now know that effective therapists do in fact share their lives with the children they treat.

Approximately 20 years after their last contact, which occurred when Cynthia called during her freshman year of college to say things were going very well, Bob was giving a presentation sponsored by a parents' group in a neighboring town. The topic was "Raising Resilient Children and Teens." At the conclusion of the talk, a number of parents came up to chat with him. A woman handed him her business card and at first Bob wondered why. Much to his surprise and delight, it was Cynthia who said, "It's what you were talking about tonight. Even troubled kids can turn out to be successful adults."

And then she added, "I'll never forget that you came to my game. It meant so much to me that you saw me doing something that I was good at."

Bob said, "I want to thank you for inviting me to the game. It influenced the way I do therapy. It helped me to realize the importance of discussing with kids and adults I see in therapy what they enjoy doing and what they see as their strengths."

Cynthia waited until other parents had finished talking with Bob. She told him that she had moved back to the area the previous year and was married and raising two children. From the information on the card she handed Bob, he could see that she had an executive coaching position with a business group.

A valuable lesson from Michael. We have developed a number of strategies to engage children to think about the events in their lives in different ways. We have come to realize that how we view an event and the words we choose make a powerful difference. For example, a parent may call a child "slow" in describing their behavior, yet we may describe that child as "careful." The very words we use to describe our children and their behavior play a significant role in how effective we may be in increasing their insight and helping them change their behavior.

In the course of working with children, Sam typically asks the child to describe what would comprise a "good day." This is an effort to help the child focus on positive rather than negative qualities, setting a foundation to create a plan for having a good day.

When Sam asked 11-year-old Michael this question he was surprised by the answer, "Good days are when bad things don't happen."

Sam was uncertain how to respond, but after a few moments of silence he asked Michael to explain further. Michael proceeded to describe a typical day in his life, one filled with negativity. He almost never woke up on time and finally got out of bed when his mother yelled at him; his brother picked on him; other kids did not want to sit next to him on the school bus; he was placed in a special education classroom and was far behind in a number of academic subjects; he was isolated on the playground during recess; he had limited after school activities because his homework was incomplete; finally, bedtime always came too soon for him. Michael very meticulously described his day, this despite the fact that he suffered from multiple learning disabilities, attention problems, and anxiety.

Michael concluded by saying, "So you see Dr. Sam, if none of those things happen then I would have a good day."

We can understand how Michael came to view the absence of anything positive along with the absence of anything negative, not as neutral, but as something "good." After some further discussion, Sam had an epiphany. He asked Michael what it would take to have "an excellent day."

Michael thought for a moment and responded, "An excellent day would be when nothing bad happened and we have pizza for supper."

This discussion served as an entry for Sam to help Michael shift his mindset and recognize that a good day was not just the absence of adversity but was replete with positive experiences. The well-meant efforts of his parents, teachers, and even his therapist to that point had failed to consider how negatively impacted he had been by a focus on fixing what was wrong or limiting what was adverse. In essence, Michael's thinking was dominated by the *medical model*.

A Focus on Resilience and a Resilient Mindset

Our collaboration, guided by common interests, including what we had learned from children and families, led us to focus increasingly on the concept of resilience. In the first book we co-authored, *Raising Resilient Children*, we defined resilience as "the ability to deal more effectively with stress and pressure, to cope with everyday challenges, to bounce back from disappointments, adversity, and trauma, to develop clear and realistic goals, to solve problems, to relate comfortably with others, and to treat oneself and others with respect."

In examining this definition of resilience, we asked, "How do resilient children (or adults) see the world and themselves differently from children (or adults) who are not resilient?" This was more than just an academic question. Rather, we knew that the more precisely we could identify the beliefs and behaviors of resilient individuals, the more effective we could be to develop guidelines and strategies for nurturing these qualities in our children and ourselves. We called these assumptions about ourselves and others a *resilient mindset*.

While children are born with certain attributes, such as a unique temperament that may serve to increase or decrease the likelihood of their becoming resilient, that is but one part of the story. The environment in which they develop and interact is also a strong determinant of whether a resilient mindset and behaviors emerge. For this reason, it is essential that parents and other caregivers, including teachers, coaches, and therapists, understand the characteristics of a resilient mindset and ways of nurturing this mindset in youngsters.

We have suggested that parents who successfully engage in the process of raising resilient youngsters possess an understanding that is sometimes explicit and other times intuitive of what they can do to nurture a resilient mindset and behaviors in their children. These parents follow a blueprint of important principles, ideas, and actions composed of resilience qualities in their day-to-day interactions with their children.

From the perspective of children, such qualities include experiencing empathy and empathic communication, being accepted and appreciated by others, having the opportunity to learn to solve problems and make decisions, and developing a social conscience. In writing about these qualities, we have defined not only the steps necessary for parents to successfully implement the teaching of these ways of thinking and behaving, but also the obstacles that often prevent well-intentioned parents, teachers, and therapists from helping their children.

We have come to realize that among the most important of these obstacles is the strong impediment that emerges when children lack effective self-discipline and parents are at a loss as to how to instill this ability in their children. In fact, all of these resilient qualities mean little if children lack the necessary self-discipline to put them into effective practice. That is, knowing what to do (e.g., possessing empathy) does not guarantee that children will do what they know (e.g., act on that feeling of empathy toward others) absent the necessary self-discipline to do so.

There is another important point we wish to emphasize that arose from our collaboration. Research related to the concept of resilience has typically focused on individuals who have faced and overcome great adversity in their lives. Studying this population is certainly understandable. However, we proposed that the research findings with at-risk populations that have produced important data about resilience should be applied to parenting practices with all children, whether or not they have faced substantial hardships.

We adopted this position for two main reasons. First, one can never predict when a child or adult may suddenly face adversity. If difficult situations should arise, then children and adults possessing a resilient mindset with its accompanying behaviors will be in a better position to effectively manage these challenges. Second, possessing a resilient mindset leads to behaviors that contribute to a less stressful, more satisfying, meaningful, and hopeful life even when individuals have been fortunate not to have encountered many obstacles.

Nurturing Islands of Competence

An essential shift from a medical to a resilience model necessitated our moving the spotlight from pathology to strengths or what we call *islands of competence*. In the beginning of our careers when we met with parents and/or teachers of children with whom we were conducting an evaluation or engaging in psychotherapy, we would spend much of the time asking about the problems, weaknesses, and vulnerabilities of the child rather than the latter's interests and strengths. The questions we posed for the children themselves were also tilted toward pathology. We began by asking what was wrong.

It seemed reasonable to center our discussion on a child's deficits since these problems were often the impetus for parents contacting us. Little did we appreciate that spending an inordinate amount of time discussing what was wrong with the child—even with the best intentions of helping that child—reinforced negative emotions and pessimism among them and the adults in their lives.

As we became increasingly aware of the shortcomings of a deficit model, we began to wonder what would happen if after just several minutes of discussing a child's problems, we would ask parents and teachers what they viewed as the child's interests and strengths. Or, what would happen if we asked children we were seeing for an evaluation or in therapy a similar question? In considering these questions, we were aware that if we placed a spotlight on strengths it must not be seen as minimizing or avoiding a child's problems.

This prompted us to say to parents and teachers, "It's important to identify your child's (student's) problems if we are to address them. However, now that we've discussed some of your child's (student's) struggles, we think it will be helpful if you could tell us what you view as your child's (student's) strengths or what we call their *islands of competence*. We've found that identifying and reinforcing the strengths of children encourages them to confront and overcome problems they face."

Relatedly, we asked children and adolescents what they judged to be their *islands of competence*. If they said they were uncertain, we replied, "That's okay, it can take time to figure out what you're good at, but it's important to do so." We immediately witnessed the benefits of asking questions about a child's strengths. A consideration of a child's *islands of competence* welcomed in a sense of hope and created positive emotions. This invited adults to be more creative in designing and implementing strategies that paved the way for youngsters to begin to identify their strengths and to deal effectively with problematic areas in their lives.

"I like the bushes better than I like school." Gavin, a 10-year-old boy, holds a special place in Bob's transition to a strength-based, therapeutic approach. When Bob made the decision to ask the next child he evaluated about their islands of competence, Gavin turned out to be that child. Gavin was referred to Bob because of his seemingly unprovoked physical aggression toward other students. The principal of Gavin's school also informed Bob that another problematic behavior occurring with greater frequency was Gavin rushing off the bus at the beginning of the school day to hide behind the bushes.

The principal told Bob that the school had attempted a point system to modify Gavin's behavior, but it proved unsuccessful. He also explained that Gavin had learning problems, which he knew intensified his dislike of school. Bob was prepared to ask Gavin about his strengths during their first meeting, but Gavin had another agenda.

Immediately upon entering our office, Gavin shouted, "I know why we're meeting!"

Bob asked, "Why?"

Gavin replied, "I hide behind the bushes of the school. I like the bushes better than I like school. What the hell do you think you're going to do about it?"

Bob was taken aback by Gavin's frank and intense pronouncement and quickly decided not to enter into a debate about bushes versus school. Instead, Bob returned to what he was going to originally ask Gavin, "If you like we can talk about bushes and school later, but what I'm always interested in when I speak with kids is what they like to do, what they think they do rather well."

This comment seemed to disarm Gavin and throw him off the path he had been taking. To Bob's pleasant surprise Gavin replied, "I like to take care of my pet dog."

Bob said, "I'm not an expert on taking care of dogs. What are some of the most important things to do when you take care of a pet dog?"

This question prompted Gavin to speak almost nonstop for the rest of the session about what to do so that pets felt you cared about them. Bob could not help thinking that Gavin was also sharing information about what Bob and others should do to help him to feel more comfortable.

Bob complimented Gavin about all of his wisdom about pets and asked if he could inform the school principal of Gavin's knowledge. The latter said it would be okay with him. When the session ended, Gavin smiled and uttered words Bob will never forget, "Good session, doc."

Shortly after the session, Bob contacted the principal and discussed appointing Gavin the pet monitor of the school. The next day, the principal called after meeting with Gavin, noting, "I like this strength-based approach. I just had a great meeting with Gavin. I told him that a class had just gotten a pet rabbit and that other classes had pets as well. I said that I was pretty certain that each class that had a pet took care of the pet. However, I wanted to have one student in the school who would check to make sure all of the pets were well taken care of. I said we could start with the rabbit."

The principal continued, "To make it even more official I laminated a 'union card' with the title of 'Pet Monitor Union' on the top. I've never seen Gavin so happy. I also spoke with Gavin's teacher about somehow using what you call his island of competence to help him feel more comfortable in school."

Gavin's teacher approached him to say that she heard how knowledgeable he was about pets. She told him, "I checked the school library and there's not a book about taking care of pets. Perhaps you could write a small book."

"I have trouble writing. I don't like to write."

His teacher responded, "That's okay, one of the reasons I became a teacher is to help my students who may have trouble learning to find new ways of learning. I would love to help you with writing your book." Gavin agreed.

Gavin was soon ensuring that all of the pets at the school were being treated kindly. With his teacher's assistance, he wrote a short book about taking care of pets and the book was bound and placed in the school library. In addition, by the end of the year he had given a brief "lecture" in every classroom about taking care of pets.

Very importantly, Gavin's aggression toward his peers and hiding behind the bushes ceased to occur. As Gavin's confidence blossomed he shared with Bob an impressive insight while they were discussing the positive changes in his behavior.

"I used to think it was better hitting another kid and be sent to the principal's office or hide behind the bushes than be in the classroom where I felt like a dummy."

Gavin's comment captured the desperate coping strategies that many children and teens employ to avoid feeling inadequate, especially in front of their peers. Unfortunately, as in Gavin's case, some of these coping strategies are self-defeating, exacerbating rather than improving a child's problems. These adverse strategies typically develop when children lose their Intuitive Optimism and Intrinsic Motivation, two key instincts of *Tenacity*. In the next chapter, we will explain and elaborate on these instincts. We often wonder what would have occurred in psychotherapy if Bob had not immediately asked Gavin about his strengths or if Gavin had not had a teacher and school principal who possessed the courage to change a punitive school approach to one that identified, honored, and displayed a challenging student's islands of competence.

The Impact of a Charismatic Adult: "You Just Have to Know My Dad"

Gavin's story as well as the others in this chapter capture a basic finding in the resilience literature; namely, resilience is rooted in the relationships that children have with caring, supportive adults. In the absence of such relationships, it is difficult for a child to become hopeful and resilient. As the late Psychologist Julius Segal, whose work focused on factors that assisted children to overcome adversity, eloquently noted:

> From studies conducted around the world, researchers have distilled a number of factors that enable such children of misfortune to beat the heavy odds against them. One factor turns out to be the presence in their lives of a charismatic adult—a person from whom they can gather strength.

We have learned that any adult can serve as a charismatic person to a child. We have been impressed by stories of parents, teachers, coaches, even neighbors providing this support.

We have introduced many techniques and strategies to better understand the thoughts and mindsets of children. One of the questions we ask children during the course of our initial interview is: If they could be anyone for a day whom would they choose? We found that children typically choose music, television, movie, or sports personalities. This question is used as an entry to help children think about their current lives and where they hope to be in the future. But 13-year-old Robert was to surprise Sam with his response.

Robert was a child with significant learning and social problems. He had few friends and was quite lonely. Without hesitation in response to Sam's question Robert responded, "My dad. You just have to know my dad. He loves me." Despite Robert's challenges, his powerful connection with his father, as displayed in his response to this question, helped us understand that regardless of the challenges or adversity this young man would face, his family connection was a powerful buffer and support. Such a connection with a caring adult has been repeatedly demonstrated to assist children with challenges to transition successfully into adulthood.

Why This Book? Why a Focus on *Tenacity*?

We noted earlier in this chapter that after co-authoring several books about the concept of resilience, we recognized that one of the components of resilience, self-discipline, deserved special consideration, leading us to write *Raising a Self-Disciplined Child*. Since that time, our thinking about resilience and self-discipline has evolved and led us to introduce in this book a third major concept—tenacity. As we have described and will further explain in detail in the next chapter, we view the seven instincts of *Tenacity* as framing our beliefs and providing the fuel for our emotions and thoughts to help us be resilient and achieve self-discipline.

In the chapters that follow, we will define what we mean by *instincts* with a focus on the seven instincts of *Tenacity*, the science examining each of these instincts, and strategies for nurturing these instincts in our children as well as in ourselves. As we have done in our previous work, we will also make note of obstacles that can derail good efforts. Additionally we will introduce and discuss three instincts that over tens of thousands of years enhanced our survival but today if left unchecked contribute to many of the challenges we and our children face. We will offer a framework for the application of the seven affirmative instincts in reducing the risk of these three.

We believe that the *essential triad of human development*—resilience, self-discipline, and tenacity—offer not just a different way of raising children and managing ourselves, but a better way. Our role as parents, educators, and therapists is not solely to teach, but to create everyday experiences that nurture these seven instincts to blossom in our children, students, and patients. We think you will agree.

Chapter 2
Tenacity is Instinctual

"Knowledge is power" wrote philosopher Sir Francis Bacon. As a word of caution, Historian Dan Boorstein wrote, "The greatest obstacle to discovery is not ignorance – it is the illusion of knowledge." How much do we really know about child development? How much of what transpires during the formative years shaping and molding our children's lives is driven by genes and instinct, acquired knowledge, or some combination of both?

Whether designed by a higher Creator or the product of millions of years of evolution, our genes have but one primary goal. They seek to continue their existence. To do so successfully requires them to transition from an older body into a younger body through the process of procreation. Our genes are resilient and indomitable. Each of us carries genes as well as bits and pieces of genes from our ancestors and their ancestors, passing back through thousands of species and millions if not billions of years.

We know little about the purpose of some of these genes nor their reason for hitchhiking in our genome. Our genes play a significant role in shaping who we are and who we become. As we have discussed, this process is dependent not only on our genes but also on our experiences and the many opportunities we have throughout our lives to acquire knowledge.

Whether the product of a benevolent Creator or a lengthy process of evolution or both matters little in our discussion. What matters is that the more complex a species (and we are among the most complex of all species on earth), the longer it takes for our young to progress to adulthood and the more important experience becomes in shaping how our genes express themselves. In genetics, this is referred to as multi-finality. Similar genes may lead to different outcomes based upon the organism's experiences. We noted in Chapter 1 that if you do not speak to children they may have all the genes to communicate but will never speak. If humans or any species never have the opportunity to socialize, despite possessing all the genes to do so, they will not be social.

© Springer Nature Switzerland AG 2021
S. Goldstein and R. B. Brooks, *Tenacity in Children*,
https://doi.org/10.1007/978-3-030-65089-6_2

How Do They Know?

Did you ever wonder why babies quickly develop a social smile and look you in the eyes? Is it surprising to learn that the muscles in your ears are set within the range of women's voices at birth or that babies prefer looking at women's faces versus men? Seeing a baby ignites rapid brain activity. In fact, researchers at the Institute of Child Health and Development find that the "cuteness" we associate with babies may help to facilitate well-being and complex social relationships by activating brain networks associated with emotion and pleasure as well as triggering empathy and compassion. In a seventh of a second, the orbitofrontal part of our brain becomes active at the sight of a baby. This rapid activity may partly explain how babies of any species appropriate our attention so quickly and completely.

What is the force behind these phenomena? The answer is a single word—instinct! It is our contention that in complex species instincts serve a critical role in shaping the developmental course through childhood into adulthood. Tens of thousands of generations of children allowed for many genetic mutations, some of which were adaptive. Some of these increased the likelihood that babies would survive, even thrive throughout their childhood, and transition successfully into adult life. Babies are born completely helpless. They are not salmon or snakes ready at birth to survive solely by relying on their instincts. They require more than a single parent like bear cubs or just a few years in a family group like gorillas, until they are ready to transition into adulthood. In our world today, we have continued to extend childhood. Some parents have observed that their children do not grow up until they are thirty!

Does an infant decide that a particular female will care for and protect her during her most vulnerable years? Is a young child aware that if he just keeps making noises eventually he will speak? Why does a toddler keep scribbling until eventually she draws or writes something meaningful? Do children know that if they just stand up, no matter how many times they fall down, they will eventually walk?

Tenacity is composed of seven instincts we will articulate in detail in this book. We consider one of the most important to be Intuitive Optimism. This is the unspoken belief that if you just keep at a task your chances of success are greater. We would argue that when it comes to reaching developmental milestones continued effort nearly always leads to success as long as the task is within the capacities of the child to achieve. This instinct is clearly a vital component of self-discipline and a resilient mindset.

Our children are in fact hard wired to learn if we are sufficiently knowledgeable to understand how their wiring interacts with the world around them and create environments in which they can grow and thrive. Every society places expectations upon its youth to acquire a certain level of knowledge and behavior in order to functionally transition into adulthood. No matter how simple the society, children must harness their instincts to acquire knowledge, develop self-discipline, cope well with adversity, and persist even in the face of failure. The instincts comprising *Tenacity* provide the critical foundation for children in any culture or society to acquire necessary knowledge to transition successfully into adult life.

A Preschool Dropout

Susan Miller's first words to us as she entered our office was, "My daughter Amy would be a preschool drop out if there was such a thing!"

Susan's smile disarmed our worry as it was clear she was starting this conversation with humor. As had become our process of history taking, we quickly asked about Amy's strengths. "My daughter is bright, can already read, and is so much fun," Susan answered.

With that, she removed a photograph from her purse and showed it to us. The photograph portrayed a line of young children, boys and girls, outdoors in a park with parents and others looking on. Susan explained that this was Amy's preschool graduation. Along with Susan, we chuckled as only the past few generations of children even attended preschool. We looked down the row of bright faces in the photograph singing a series of songs they had dutifully rehearsed. These youngsters possessed the memory to learn the songs, the self-discipline to stand and sing each song, and the respect for their teacher to sing when requested.

We asked, "Which one of these girls is your daughter?" Susan didn't respond immediately but explained that this was her daughter's third preschool in two years. "You see," Susan explained, "My daughter is not a good pre-school executive. Oh, she is smart but scattered. She can't keep track of her crayons, there are only two left in her box. She also can't seem to keep her bottom on the assigned carpet square during story time and wanders the room. Suffice it to say teachers think she doesn't try hard enough to follow the rules."

This pattern of a lack of fit between Amy's temperament and her ability to regulate herself to the preschool teacher's expectation wasn't new to us. We had worked with hundreds of families raising children with a challenging temperament. We looked closely at the photograph but still couldn't discern the "problem child."

Susan continued. "You can stop looking. Amy is not in that photograph." This worried us. What was Amy's great crime? Why had she had been excluded from this important event? Before we could inquire further, Susan produced another photograph of a hillside about fifty yards behind and to the right of the group. There on top of the hill, waving to her mother was Amy! She had wandered away with little notice. Susan had the insight to take a photograph before chasing up the hill to retrieve her daughter.

We don't want to pathologize, demonize, nor moralize Amy's challenges. Assigning a label and setting out to fix Amy may keep her in line and her bottom on the carpet square but does it truly prepare Amy to successfully transition through chiildhood. We think, as we have written, that symptom relief is valuable but only the first step in raising resilient, self-disciplined, tenacious children. Amy will require her parents and educators to understand the seven instincts of *Tenacity* and patiently find ways to foster and grow them in Amy. For Amy, progress may be slow, but slow will be fast enough.

The Role of Parents

For thousands of generations, parents, relatives, and the extended community raised and prepared children to become successful adults, to acquire knowledge and strengthen the abilities needed to meet the challenges of their time. How did they do it? Until relatively recent times in human history, there were no schools or organized institutions, nor were there self-help or parenting books. We believe the foundation of this process was accomplished by caregivers drawing upon seven important instincts in their offspring that have evolved over tens if not hundreds of thousands of years in ours and other hominid species.

In some species, instincts are fixed patterns of behavior leading to a certain outcome such as a bird building a nest for the first time or a salmon returning upriver to its birthplace to spawn. We believe that in our species instincts represent an intuitive way of thinking and/or acting that increase the chances of survival and success. In viewing instincts in this way we appreciate that knowing what to do and doing what you know are not synonymous and are very much dependent on experience. These instincts are more important than ever in preparing today's children for tomorrow's successes.

Our book is a roadmap for parents, teachers, coaches, mentors, and all adults committed to providing all children with the opportunity to access, strengthen, and employ these instincts as they negotiate childhood and journey into adult life. The instincts comprising *Tenacity* furnish the power to build self-discipline and resilience. For these instincts to develop and flourish, they require the nurturing and support of caring, knowledgeable adults. In short, it is our job to help children harness the power of their instincts.

The Seven Instincts of *Tenacity*

Parents effectively engaging in the processes necessary to foster and reinforce these instincts possess an implicit, explicit, or even intuitive understanding of how they can help their children acquire self-discipline and a resilient mindset. In our first book, *Raising Resilient Children*, we suggested that capable parents' guide their interactions with children through a blueprint of important principles, ideas, and actions. We pointed out that grasping the complexities of this blueprint is an ongoing process filled with challenges, frustrations, setbacks, and successes.

We have come to appreciate that there is much variability housed in this blueprint of knowledge, ideas, and actions; a blueprint that to be effective requires modification for each child. Though you may wish for the one true, golden path to your children's future, such a path doesn't exist. However, understanding the role of these seven instincts will comfort and provide you with the knowledge to help your children. While the path to adulthood is shaped by countless factors including your children's temperament, family style and values, educational and social experiences, and the broader society and culture in which you raise children, the principles and ideas of these instincts are universal and applicable to everyone. The remainder of this chapter briefly introduces each of these seven instincts and begins to describe the ways in which each influences development.

The seven instincts of *Tenacity* are:

1. Intuitive Optimism
2. Intrinsic Motivation
3. Compassionate Empathy
4. Simultaneous Intelligence
5. Genuine Altruism
6. Virtuous Responsibility
7. Measured Fairness.

Let's get acquainted with each of these instincts and the knowledge required to help children bring them "online."

1. **Intuitive Optimism**

Intuitive Optimism, which we introduced earlier in this chapter, can be defined as "born believing." The more complex the species, the longer the time taken to mature, the more tasks to be mastered, the more important it is to believe success or a goal is attainable. Intuitive implies that children do not have to learn by experience alone, they just know. Optimism implies that no matter what challenge comes before them they retain the belief that with necessary caregiver assistance and their own perseverance they will ultimately experience success.

Intuitive Optimism explains why children absent any knowledge of their capacity or potential for success are willing to try again and again to master developmental tasks. All children come into the world with some degree of Intuitive Optimism. It is the engine that drives their daily quest to understand and master the world around them. Intuitive Optimism is a core component in a child's resilient mindset. Resilience as we have written is a pattern of positive adjustment and adaptation in the context of any challenge or adversity. Resilient children harness their Intuitive Optimism to persevere time and time again.

We fondly remember a conversation with Andy, a precocious six-year-old boy. Andy explained that he wanted his dad to buy the neighbor's old car so he, Andy, could "make it into a race car." We asked if Andy had ever fixed a car. Andy quickly and confidently responded, "No, but Dad can teach me and I can do it!" We smile at young children's Intuitive Optimism. They believe they can cook, fix anything, and drive the car! Some adults think these beliefs are an example of childish immaturity. We believe these ideas represent the sometime humorous but essential manifestations of Intuitive Optimism.

2. **Intrinsic Motivation**

Intrinsic Motivation is best defined as motivation from the inside out. It is rooted in the joy of engaging and eventually succeeding at a task. It is not derived from coercive, punitive, or reward-driven parenting but from creating opportunities for children, even at young ages, to experience pleasure when they are involved in activities that generate excitement and pleasure. Their reward is built into doing the task.

Can you imagine a situation in which a young child asked a parent for a reward in exchange for playing in the sandbox? Seems absurd. However, think about this, you quickly realize that children's curiosity driven by their Intuitive Optimism is all the reward or reinforcement they require to engage in everyday activities. Young children engage in activities not because they are receiving external or extrinsic motivators, but because they simply enjoy the activity and/or the activity provides them with an opportunity to help. After all, up until just recent times, everyone in a family or tribal group, regardless of age, was required to help out.

More than 50 years ago, Harvard Psychologist, Dr. Robert White advanced the belief that there is an inborn need or motivation in children to be effective individuals and to master the challenges they will face in their future environment. The combination of Intuitive Optimism and Intrinsic Motivation explains why the majority of children embrace the concept of school. Parents often comment that their young children can't wait to go to school at the beginning of the new school year. Sometimes they believe it's because older siblings attend school or the child has the opportunity to wear new clothes or to ride the school bus. However Intrinsic Motivation plays a large role.

Sadly, this enthusiasm is quickly dampened for some children. They soon learn that the school environment is one in which you will be judged and evaluated in a competitive atmosphere: an atmosphere in which no matter how well you perform you will repeatedly be reminded there is always room for improvement. Children initially embrace school because it presents yet another developmental challenge they are intuitively optimistic they will master and are intrinsically motivated to engage in. Yet, the first thing that happens when children enter school is they encounter an educational system all-too-often driven by a stimulus–response model that offers the promise of a reward, the threat of a punishment, or the challenge of a competition in an effort to motivate them.

These three extrinsic motivators may seem at first to be effective but at a steep price. They very clearly work against and challenge the continued nurturance and development of Intrinsic Motivation, that is, succeeding at school for the sheer pleasure and enjoyment of success and learning. The belief that effort is not in the service of obtaining high grades, money, or privileges but rather because accomplishment itself is intrinsically motivating is soon eclipsed by the promise of external rewards.

Unfortunately, when children with learning, emotional, behavioral, social, academic, or other developmental problems enter school, they quickly begin to struggle. Struggling at school is often defined as being too slow or not trying hard enough. Our educational system has determined that these struggles require a greater degree of extrinsic motivation to keep children involved in school activities. The more challenges children experience in school, the more extrinsic rewards are provided for the additional effort these children must exert. Yet it is exactly these students who require more of our diligence to ensure that we do not steal or chip away at their intrinsic motivation when they struggle in school.

We are not proposing elimination of grades, rewards, punishments, or competitions in our educational system, but that for all students and especially those who struggle, we must be mindful of keeping a balance between the use of extrinsic motivators and the continued nurturance of intrinsic motivation. Far too often, the balance is skewed toward extrinsic rewards. Yet, it is Intrinsic Motivation that drives self-reinforcement, a phenomenon that we believe strongly is the foundation of life success and happiness, even more important than intellect, ability, and opportunity.

3. Compassionate Empathy

Empathy is the ability to understand the world of others on both cognitive and affective levels. Compassion is perceived of as calling upon that understanding to initiate actions that express caring toward others.

Imagine for a moment what your relationships with others would be like if you constantly struggled to understand their perspective. Imagine not being able to decipher accurately what others are feeling or communicating. Think about a time you were in a situation in which you felt you could not "read" the other person, could not sense their intentions nor what they were experiencing. What if you were coming across in a manner that was upsetting to other people but you did not comprehend why they seemed to be annoyed or upset by your behavior, or you did not even realize they were upset?

Compassionate Empathy is an essential component of emotional and social intelligence. Compassionate Empathy facilitates effective communication and allows our children to understand how much we care about and love them. It permits us to be more effective disciplinarians as we teach our children values. Modeling and teaching Compassionate Empathy help children develop social competence, knowledge they can skillfully apply in their relationships throughout their lives.

It often appears that children with Autism Spectrum Disorder come into the world limited in this instinct and in their capacity to strengthen and grow this instinct through experience. We know however from our experiences that even children with Autism Spectrum Disorder can develop and strengthen Compassionate Empathy if we understand what they require from us. In fact, we authored a book for parents *Raising Resilient Children with Autism Spectrum Disorders* that included strategies for reinforcing empathy in children with this diagnosis.

It is often challenging to be empathic with our children even when they do not struggle with learning, behavior, or socialization. The challenge is magnified appreciably when parenting a child who displays such problems. It is difficult to place one's self inside the shoes of a child whose perceptions and behaviors are often strikingly different from our own. We will address this issue in Chapter 5.

4. Simultaneous Intelligence

Simultaneous Intelligence guides our practical understanding of how elements of a problem fit together into a solution. Simultaneous Intelligence at its core is the process of reasoning and critically thinking to solve problems. This instinct is not culture or experience bound. For two thousand years, intelligence was defined as how well you solved problems, not how well you could read or write, or the number of years you attended school. After all, education as an undeniable right is a late nineteenth-century idea. Unfortunately, the advent of mandatory education 150 years ago has led intelligence to be largely defined as the extent to which a child possesses a body of knowledge. Even today, many schools require advanced academic achievement or acquired knowledge along with strong Simultaneous Intelligence to qualify for gifted education.

Current conceptualizations of intelligence have been widely debated. Historically, intelligence tests have been demonstrated as a good predictor of school achievement. Up until recently, intelligence tests were very content heavy. However, these tests are relatively similar to those that measure achievement. As such, there has been a lack of distinction between current measures of intelligence and achievement, resulting in disadvantages for those who have not adequately received strong educational experiences and opportunities at home and/or in their early years.

The lack of distinction between academic knowledge and intelligence is the driving factor that results in individuals with low socioeconomic status obtaining lower intellectual scores on many tests used in our schools. It is important for us to move beyond the reliance of acquired academic knowledge in our understanding of intelligence. It is essential that we develop a model based on understanding the ways in which a child or for that matter all of us processes information, reasons, and solves problems. Simultaneous Intelligence offers such a framework.

5. Genuine Altruism

Altruism is an unselfish concern for and support of the survival of others. Genuine Altruism is most synonymous with what might be considered as pure altruism. It is the giving of yourself with no expectation of a return for your actions. We help others achieve their goals even when the helper receives no immediate benefit and the person helped is a stranger. Genuine Altruism is rare among nearly all species and may be a uniquely human instinct. Researchers have demonstrated that children as young as 18 months old will readily help others to achieve their goals. This form of helping others without reciprocity is strongly driven by Compassionate Empathy as well as related to Virtuous Responsibility and Measured Fairness, which we will discuss below. Researchers Drs. Felix Warneken and Michael Tomasello have demonstrated Genuine Altruism in a variety of ways with very young children and even chimpanzees! We will visit their research in Chapter 7.

6. Virtuous Responsibility

We have noticed an alarming trend in the news in the past few years. American President Harry Truman, of the buck stops here fame, would "roll over in his grave" if he could. Everyone appears equally guilty of this behavior regardless of wealth, ethnicity, or political affiliation. It seems that fewer and fewer people take responsibility for their actions and behavior. In light of what they constantly see reported in the media, it is not surprising that the most frequent comment from the youth with whom we work is "it's not my fault." Where have we gone wrong? How can we expect children to act responsibly when they are repeatedly confronted by adults who do not?

Virtue is about principles and ethics. Responsibility is about being accountable for your actions. However, Virtuous Responsibility is more than just accepting culpability or blame, a narrow view that would deprive this instinct of its powerful positive meaning. This instinct involves meeting responsibilities that protect and enrich one's society. Harvard Government Professor Michael Sandel, during a 2020 interview with Leigh Wells that examined each citizen's responsibilities during The COVID-19 pandemic, observed, "Our ethical obligations are, first of all, to minimize the possibility that our behavior will expose others to the risk of contracting the virus. Beyond this, those of us who are fortunate enough to work from the safety of our homes have a responsibility to support those who take risks on our behalf."

This broader view of Virtuous Responsibility captures how closely related it is to the instincts of Compassionate Empathy and Intrinsic Motivation. As noted earlier, young children possess an inborn need to be helpful. They take great pleasure when engaged in what we have called contributory activities as is evident in their bright smiles when their actions are complimented and appreciated. These contributory activities are displayed during each and every day. They want to help us cook, take care of younger siblings, rake leaves, mow the lawn, build with our tools, sweep the kitchen, and set the table. Through opportunities to act responsibly, children learn to accept and embrace the consequences of their actions even when they fail or make mistakes. By helping children develop Virtuous Responsibility, we are helping them reach their full potential. But we must remember that Virtuous Responsibility goes beyond helping others. It eventually involves making decisions, being trusted, and learning to be accountable for one's actions—whether these actions result in positive or negative outcomes.

Though the current scientific research is not as strong in providing the instinctual foundation for Virtuous Responsibility, we believe given our experiences with thousands of children and families that opportunity and even instruction while essential alone will not lead to responsible behavior. We believe children possess an instinctual need or drive to act responsibly and when given the opportunity will make a positive difference in the lives of others. While many children can be self-centered at times, placing their own needs first, this trait is often accompanied simultaneously by a pattern in which they achieve pleasure in reaching out and enriching the lives of others.

We reported this dynamic when we described Gavin in Chapter 1. His stated interest and skills in taking care of his dog led to his being recruited as the pet monitor of the school. Shining the light on his *island of competence* and asking him to contribute to the well-being of pets and share his knowledge with his peers had a noticeable impact. His behavior and learning improved significantly.

We are aware that many parents report that their children's early desire to help and be responsible seems to diminish by the middle childhood years. They resist many opportunities to be of assistance unless there is something in it for them. However, we have observed that the expression of Virtuous Responsibility for many children does not wane but instead is shifted to helping and being responsible to friends. We often tell parents that the fact that their children now display responsibility toward their peer group indicates that the parents did a good job reinforcing this instinct in their children.

In our book *Raising Resilient Children*, we closely linked the development of responsibility, compassion, and a social conscience. We still believe these concepts are closely related, but that they deserve to be delineated further. The instinct of Virtuous Responsibility guides the emergence of responsible behavior and reinforces the expression of Compassionate Empathy and a social conscience. As children develop this foundation, which are a key component of a resilient mindset, a commitment to be accountable for one's life emerges. Responsible children and adults are more likely to accept accountability for their behavior in an honest, open manner. Such acceptance allows them to learn and initiate more positive, prosocial forms of behavior.

7. Measured Fairness

The instinct of Measured Fairness lies at the fundamental level of our social selves. This world and the many species in it evolved and survived because of this instinct. For thousands of generations being fair to others in your family or tribe ensured everyone's survival. Everyone contributed equally. And so, fairness has its nemesis: unfairness. How many times have you heard "But that's not fair" from your children? How many times have you said those words? Why do we care so much about fairness? Why does it bother us so much? Has your child ever felt an injustice? Has he spoken to you about being bullied or watched as someone jumps in front of the lunch line but everyone was afraid to say anything? We all live with varying degrees of injustice or unfairness. We manage as best we can. In fact, we've seen others who are "managing" in painful or destructive ways. We can help our children do better.

How does anyone find the path back from injustice? How do you bounce back from unfairness, whether it's caused by minor day-to-day interactions with people or an unthinkable, tragic event? For anyone who has been on the receiving end of an unfair act, you know the deep emotions associated with it. We often find the behavior intolerable and seek understanding or even retribution. Some people will even spend a life's savings in litigation fees simply to prove a point, right a wrong.

As important as examining how we find the path back from injustice, we should ask what are the best ways for nurturing the instinct of Measured Fairness in our children? We will explore these in Chapter 9.

Our Children, Their Future

Children come into this world with different temperaments and other inborn attributes. Like diamonds, no two are exactly alike. However, all are genetically endowed to some extent with the seven instincts of *Tenacity*. It is our charge as shepherds of the next generation to nurture and develop these instincts in all children regardless of their temperament, behavior, achievement, or development. These seven instincts form the lifelong foundation of a resilient mindset and effective self-discipline. Subsequent chapters will explore and define the strategies required to foster and enhance these instincts in every child and in doing so, ourselves.

Chapter 3
Intuitive Optimism

Larry, a 24-month-old toddler, is building a tower of wooden blocks. A look of glee crosses his face as he stacks one block on top of another glancing at his delighted parents as he does so. As the tower gets taller, it becomes increasingly unstable, but Larry persists. As he places one more block on top, the tower topples over and the blocks scatter on the floor. He looks bewildered, perhaps surprised that the tower fell over.

Before his parents can say or do anything, Larry says "Me do" and proceeds to rebuild the tower. He even accepts his mother's assistance as she straightens the blocks so that the tower becomes sturdier. However, before long this taller tower also crashes to the ground.

Larry once again asserts "Me do" and begins the building process for a third time with the glee returning to his face.

Although one has to be careful not to attribute more meaning to Larry's actions than may be warranted, his persistence is obvious. We believe that the display of such determination accompanied by a seemingly joyful demeanor captures the instinct of Intuitive Optimism, a belief that happier and successful endings can be achieved.

Contrast Larry's behavior with that of Eli. His parents contacted us when Eli was 6 years old, worried about how easily he became frustrated when he faced setbacks and obstacles, whether learning to ride a two-wheel bicycle, attempting to hit a ball, or learning to recite the alphabet. They reported that his typical response in such situations was to quit, saying the task was "stupid" or "boring." Or, depending on the activity, he would sometimes blame them or others. In addition, they were concerned that he often refused to attempt new activities. They surmised that he did not believe he could succeed. Eli seemed impervious to their words of encouragement. "It's as if he chooses to be unhappy," they told us, perplexed by Eli's seeming resistance to change.

We asked Eli's parents if these worrisome behaviors were relatively new. They responded no and immediately recalled that when Eli was just 24 months old he would become frustrated when building a tower with blocks. When the blocks fell over, Eli would pick them up and throw them against the wall, shouting, "Bad blocks."

© Springer Nature Switzerland AG 2021

S. Goldstein and R. B. Brooks, *Tenacity in Children*,

https://doi.org/10.1007/978-3-030-65089-6_3

Eli's mother said, "He was so young, but it was if a pattern was being established, blaming other things or people for mistakes. After a few attempts he wouldn't build with the blocks anymore, even when we offered to help him."

Consider these two 24-month-old children, one whose behavior reflected that he believed that better outcomes existed in the future, the other sensing continued failure. One optimistic, one not, yet both had caring parents. Although in the last chapter we advanced the position that Intuitive Optimism is instinctual, Eli's behavior at such a young age might suggest otherwise. However, we still hold that position, which leads to two other ideas that are not only applicable to Intuitive Optimism but also to the six other instincts, namely: Although a behavior may be instinctual, complex human instincts require multiple factors, including a child's inborn temperament and early life experiences, to shape the behaviors associated with that instinct in order to flourish.

There are many strategies that parents and other caregivers can employ to strengthen all of the seven instincts and, if necessary, provide a new path when the nurturance of an instinct has been derailed in the normal course of development.

What is Intuitive Optimism?

As described in Chapter 2, Intuitive Optimism may be defined as "born believing." The word "intuitive" implies that children do not have to learn by experience alone. They just know. "Optimism" suggests that regardless of the challenges they face, they retain the belief that with perseverance they will ultimately experience success. It was this instinct that propelled Larry to continue to build a tower of blocks with obvious glee even when previous attempts failed. It was a weakening of Intuitive Optimism for whatever reasons that led Eli to give up his quest for building a tower and to subsequently blame the blocks for toppling over.

Optimism has been studied and conceptualized in different ways. It is valuable to spend time in the beginning of this chapter considering these ideas. Dr. Christopher Peterson, Professor of Psychology at the University of Michigan, observed, "Contemporary approaches usually treat optimism as a cognitive characteristic—a goal, an expectation, or a causal attribution—which is sensible as long as we remember that the belief in question concerns future occurrences about which individuals have strong feelings."

In calling attention to the strong emotions that are often associated with optimism, Dr. Peterson cautioned, "Optimism is not simply cold cognition, and if we forget the emotional flavor that pervades optimism, we can make little sense of the fact that optimism is both motivated and motivating."

Psychology Professors, Drs. Michael Scheier and Charles Carver introduced the concept of *dispositional optimism*, nearly thirty years ago. They viewed this as the expectation that "good things will be plentiful in the future and bad things scarce." Their focus was on how individuals pursue goals, especially in the face of obstacles. People were seen as optimistic if they continued to strive toward goals that they perceived as attainable. They measured optimism with a brief self-report instrument called the Life Orientation Test (LOT), which included items such as:

In uncertain times, I usually expect the best.

If something can go wrong for me, it will (reverse-scored).

A group of psychologists at the University of Pennsylvania have conducted some of the most well-known research related to the concept of optimism. Drs. Karen Reivich, Jane Gilliam, Martin Seligman, and Andrew Shatte have focused their work on the study of *learned optimism*. This research is an outgrowth of Dr. Seligman's broader study of positive psychology. Initially, Dr. Seligman, who is frequently referred to as the father of positive psychology, and his co-researcher Dr. Steven Maier examined the concept of *learned helplessness* before Dr. Seligman shifted to studying *learned optimism*. These theories of helplessness and optimism are rooted in the explanatory style that people employed to interpret the causes of both negative and positive events in their lives.

A similar model was proposed by Social Psychologist Bernard Weiner over 35 years ago through his description of *attribution theory*. As an illustration, optimistic children, while giving credit to others who assisted them, viewed their successes as determined in great part by their own resources, while pessimistic children offered external reasons for any accomplishments such as: "I was lucky," "The teacher gave an easy test," "The pitcher didn't throw the ball very hard and that's why I could hit it." If you believe your success is predicated on these so-called external forces, then it is difficult to be optimistic about future success over which you have little, if any, control.

The frameworks proposed by Drs. Seligman and Weiner also examined the explanations that people chose when confronted with failure. Optimists interpreted such setbacks as situations from which they could learn rather than feel defeated. They accepted realistic help from adults and believed they could initiate new approaches to succeed.

In contrast, pessimists attributed mistakes to phenomena not amenable to change, for example, "I'm dumb," "I was born with half a brain," or "I'll never be able to do this" and our very favorite—"The teacher is dumb and doesn't know how to teach so how can I learn anything?" When harboring the kinds of thoughts that close off the promise of future accomplishment, it is not unusual for such individuals to engage in counterproductive coping strategies (e.g., quitting or rationalizing). Such strategies unfortunately exacerbate the problem.

These theories frame the instinct of Intuitive Optimism and lay the foundation for parents, educators, and therapists to develop and reinforce this instinct in children. We will review several effective strategies at a later point in this chapter.

The Benefits of Optimism

If questioned about the role of optimism in our lives, we believe most people would respond that being optimistic is important, that as Dr. Peterson wrote, optimism serves as a source of motivation to move beyond setbacks and to more confidently face new challenges. We would concur with this assessment and add that a burgeoning body of research suggests that an optimistic outlook not only prepares us to confront and overcome challenges, but in addition is a significant contributor to both our physical and emotional well-being.

Multiple research studies have demonstrated that optimistic individuals have a reduced risk of heart disease, stroke, declines in lung capacity and function, and a lower risk of early death from cancer and infection. Optimism also appears to contribute to longevity in life. In two studies completed in 2019, one involving women in which the Life Orientation Test was administered, and the other involving men in which an Optimism–Pessimism Scale was used, higher levels of optimism were associated with longevity in life. The findings of these studies are particularly important as the researchers controlled for factors such as chronic physical illness, including hypertension and high cholesterol, as well as health-related behaviors such as smoking and alcohol use. In layman terms, they made certain that none of these factors was responsible for their positive findings.

Many other studies support these affirmative findings. Not surprisingly, they conjure up images of the chicken and the egg dilemma as noted in a 2008 *Harvard Health* publication. "People who are healthy are likely to have a brighter outlook than people who are ill so perhaps optimism is actually the result of good health instead of the other way around." This is certainly a reasonable question to pose. This was examined by researchers, tracking people for 15, 30, and 40 years. The researchers concluded that "medical conditions did not tarnish the benefits of a bright outlook on life."

Another potential reason to explain the prevailing research results is that people who are optimistic are healthier and live longer than pessimists because they adhere to healthier lifestyles, nurture stronger relationships, and receive better medical care. As the Harvard article reported, "Indeed some studies report that optimists are more likely to exercise, less likely to smoke, more likely to live with a spouse, and more likely to follow medical advice than pessimists." However, optimism was "not generally associated with a better diet or leaner physique, and even when results are adjusted for cardiovascular risk factors, a beneficial effect of optimism persists."

While a more precise answer to the nature of the association between optimism and health—whether, for example, the association is causal or correlational—may not be available at this time, that should not deter us from implementing strategies to strengthen the instinct of Intuitive Optimism in our children.

Nurturing Tenacity

A number of important points must be emphasized before we offer strategies for reinforcing Intuitive Optimism as well as the six additional instincts we address in the coming chapters.

The first point may seem evident but is worth highlighting; namely, whether we desire to be or not, we are our children's first models. More than we may realize, children listen closely to what we say but are even more attuned to what we do. If we want our children to develop and strengthen the seven instincts of *Tenacity*, our daily actions must reflect an expression of these instincts.

For instance, it will be much more challenging for Intuitive Optimism (or the six other instincts) to blossom in our children if they do not witness such behaviors in their parents. Children hearing parents constantly express pessimistic thoughts (e.g., "This will never work," or "Bad things always seem to happen"), or viewing parents quit in the face of failure will have a more difficult time developing Intuitive Optimism than children whose parents display behaviors associated with optimism.

A second point, closely related to the first, is the importance of Compassionate Empathy and empathic communication in understanding and responding to children (as well as to others). We will discuss this in great depth in Chapter 5 but need to lay the foundation here. We have worked with well-meaning parents, teachers, and other caregivers who have expressed what they believe to be positive comments to children, but the comments have not been experienced as positive by the children.

We often use the following example to illustrate this point and to capture the importance of empathic communication. This involves a child being told to "try harder" when attempting to complete a certain project or to learn certain material. Parents may perceive "try harder" as conveying encouragement, but children will typically interpret those words as judgmental or accusatory. As one young adult told us, "How did they know I wasn't trying hard enough? I was having enough trouble learning and this kind of comment made things even worse." In fact, you may be surprised to learn that although we have tests to measure almost every human quality, emotion, achievement, or behavior, we do not have a test to measure how hard someone is trying!

It is for this reason that we emphasize empathic communication and ask parents and other caregivers to reflect upon the following questions when interacting with children:

"Would I want anyone to say or do to me what I have just said to my child?"

"In anything I say or do what do I hope to accomplish?"

"Am I saying or doing things in a way that would allow my children to listen to what I have to say and learn from me?"

Keeping these questions in the forefront of communications with our children will help these messages to be more effective, lessening the probability of them responding with anger or acting defensive.

Fostering Intuitive Optimism

Let's now review several strategies that form the foundation for the reinforcement of Intuitive Optimism.

Reinforce "personal control" from an early age. A central finding derived from research about optimism pertains to a concept we have highlighted in several of our previous works, namely "personal control." Optimistic people learn to focus their time and energy on situations they know they can influence rather than attempting to change situations over which they have little, if any, control. They assume what we have called a "we are the authors of our own lives" mentality. They recognize that while there are situations that arise over which they have little, if any, control, what they do have control over is their attitude and response toward those situations.

Madison was referred to us when she was nine years old. She was diagnosed with dyslexia three years earlier. Her parents, Mia and Joe Salter, reported that since the diagnosis was made, Madison had received reading assistance and was making slow but steady progress. They were especially concerned however by what they perceived to be their daughter's increasing frustration and disappointment. Just prior to the parents calling us, Madison had told her parents, "I don't know if I'll ever learn to read like the other kids," adding, "I wish I never had dyslexia. Why do I have to have it?"

Mia told us, "It's been so painful to watch Madison's distress. Her teachers and tutors have been very supportive and we've pointed out to Madison that she's made progress and shouldn't be so discouraged. We've told her about famous people with dyslexia who were very successful as adults, but she usually says she's not them."

Joe observed, "When Mia used the word 'painful,' all I could think of is that Madison always seems to give up. It appears she believes that she's a victim of dyslexia. She's thinking more about what she can't do than what she may be able to do. As Mia said, Madison's had supportive teachers and tutors and I think we've been supportive as well, but Madison doesn't seem to believe us or that things can improve."

Joe added, "I love Madison, but sometimes I find myself getting annoyed with what I consider to be her defeatist attitude. The other day I said something to her that I know I shouldn't have said, but I was just feeling so frustrated. After she told me once again that she would never learn to read like her friends and that she wished she was never born with dyslexia, I told her that as long as she had that attitude, she would have trouble learning. As soon as I said it, I knew it wasn't very helpful, especially when she started to cry and left the room."

It was evident that Mia and Joe cared deeply about Madison, were "pained" by her pessimism, and had been diligent in working with the school to obtain services for her. If you were their consultant, what might you advise them to say or do to nurture a sense of personal control and Intuitive Optimism in their daughter?

Mia and Joe's frustration and worries were understandable. A key challenge is not to permit these emotions to impact negatively on the ways in which they responded to Madison's distress. In our parent counseling sessions with Mia and Joe, we were careful to model empathy in what we said to them. An initial step was to validate their feelings, recognizing that validation need not imply agreement with another person's point of view but rather that you are attempting to understand that person's perspective.

We noted, "We can appreciate how much you care about Madison and all of your efforts to help her, not only with her reading problems, but the stress and uncertainty she feels because of these problems. And, Joe, sometimes as parents we say things that we wish we hadn't. What's important is what we can learn from this to be more empathic and helpful in the future."

Joe replied, "I'm eager to learn."

In subsequent meetings with Mia and Joe, we focused on their validating Madison's feelings and helping her gain a stronger sense of personal control, which would then reinforce their daughter's optimism. We suggested that when Madison voiced pessimism about ever learning to read effectively or fell into a victim's mentality of "why did I have to be born with dyslexia?" one way they might respond is the following:

"We know that it can be very frustrating to have trouble learning to read, especially when you see your friends learning more quickly. And, we know that it's easy to ask why did I have to be born with dyslexia? We want to say something and we hope you don't feel like we're criticizing you, since that's not what we want to do. But if you feel we are criticizing you, please let us know. We're just trying to figure out how we can be of help."

A word of caution. In this book, we offer many suggestions of what parents might say or do with their children. However, there is no precise formula or recipe. Our wording is meant as a template to illustrate, for instance, what might be said to a child with Madison's mindset. The exact words parents use should be based on the specific situation and the unique characteristics of their child.

What is the purpose of the wording we suggested to Mia and Joe? Very importantly, it validates what Madison has been asserting. Since she believes that her parents have been critical of her attitude and behaviors, the intent of the comment, "We want to say something and we hope you don't feel like we're criticizing you, since that's not what we want to do," is to prepare Madison to hear a particular opinion without having a knee-jerk negative reaction. In our experience, such preparation actually lessens the probability of a child immediately perceiving the remarks of parents as judgmental. In addition, inviting Madison to let them know if she feels they are being critical of her further reduces the possibility of an immediate negative response, while encouraging ongoing dialogue.

In our individual sessions with Madison as well as in our parent counseling meetings with Mia and Joe, we were also guided by the goal of reinforcing a sense of personal control. In our discussions with Madison, we empathized with her frustration and anger at "being born with dyslexia," adding, "Many kids who have dyslexia wonder why they had to have it. We don't know why some kids are born with dyslexia and others are not. Fortunately, we're learning more and more about ways to help kids with dyslexia learn to read. It still can be difficult, but with help it can become less of a struggle."

The essence of this comment was to convey the belief that while no one had control over Madison being born with dyslexia, what we do have control over is obtaining the best possible services for her. A portrait of optimism is rooted in our comment.

Teach problem-solving strategies. It is difficult for children to develop a sense of personal control and an optimistic outlook if their immediate response to a challenging situation is, "I don't even know where to start to deal with this problem." When this is the dominating thought, children are less likely to believe that they are authors of their own lives or that a more hopeful future lies ahead.

In many ways, children lacking problem-solving strategies feel anxious and adrift, like captains lost at sea without a compass, following one course or another but without any sound information to guide their actions. No captain would feel optimistic in such a situation.

In our previous books, we have highlighted a sequence that parents can use to help their children of any age learn to be more effective problem solvers. It is based on the work of our friend and colleague Dr. Myrna Shure. Dr. Shure was instrumental in developing the I Can Problem Solve (ICPS) program, which is described in her books *Raising a Thinking Child* and *Raising a Thinking Preteen.*

Dr. Shure advises parents not to rush in to solve their children's problems; to do so will rob them of opportunities to actively solve problems themselves. The message children may take from this parental action is "I have to rescue you because I don't think you are capable of handling the situation." Even well-meaning, loving parents who desire their children to display tenacity can easily fall into this "rescue" response.

We are aware that different situations dictate a different amount of parental input. However, parents should always assess their level of assistance and whether it will allow their children to have the experience of solving their own problems. As Dr. Shure has found, even very young children can suggest strategies for solving problems when given the platform to do so.

A guiding principle for parents when engaging their children in ways to manage various challenges is not only to resolve the issue at hand but to convey a message that reinforces a sense of personal control and optimism. Seemingly simple statements such as: "You really figured out how to do that math problem" or "That's seems like an excellent way of telling your friend how you're feeling" go a long way toward promoting tenacity.

The following sequence is one we recommend to parents, not only when interacting with their children but to use in all aspects of their lives. This three part sequence may seem very straightforward, but its application requires skill and patience if it is to be effective.

Articulate the problem and agree that it is a problem. It is difficult to solve a problem if it is not well defined. Also, while on most occasions parents and children will voice agreement that a problem exists, especially if the child is the one who brings it up, sometimes a parent may perceive the presence of a problem, but the child does not.

As a well-recognized example, many parents can think of times they asked their children to clean up their messy rooms, but (a) their children didn't view their rooms as messy or (b) even if they acknowledge they are somewhat messy, they don't see any need to clean up. In such instances, parents must find ways to explain why they see the situation as a problem but in a manner that does not evoke further annoyance and inertia.

A validating statement such as "I know that you don't see having clothes and books all over the floor as a problem, but I would like to explain why I do and then perhaps we can figure out the best way to handle things" can help to create a more cooperative, problem-solving atmosphere. The words "*we* can figure out the best way to handle things" convey a respect for the child's input, increasing the latter's sense of ownership in the process.

Consider two or three possible solutions and what the likely outcome of each will be. Once an agreement has been reached in identifying the problem, the next step is to find two or three possible solutions to solve the problem. It is during this step that many parents may find it easier and less of a hassle to suggest solutions to their children without eliciting or involving their children's input. Some children for various reasons may even welcome parents telling them what to do or have parents do something for them.

One illustration of this dynamic occurs when children passively sit back as their parents complete most of their homework for them. At that moment, everyone may experience some temporary relief as the level of stress in the home diminishes. Children and their parents have taken what seems to be the easiest, least burdensome route, but the easiest is not necessarily the best in terms of preparing children to meet the future challenges they will confront. In such a case, it will be difficult for them to develop confidence in their own abilities, leaving them vulnerable to feeling defeated when their parents are not available to assist them.

In our past writings, we have provided examples of the disadvantages of parents too quickly attempting to solve problems faced by their children. One such illustration involves nine-year-old Jane Jones who came home from school in tears. She sobbed to her mother Lilly that some of her friends refused to sit with her at lunch, telling her they did not want her around. Jane was confused and upset about her friends' rejection and asked her mother what she should do.

On the one hand, Lilly was aware of the importance of children learning to solve problems on their own or with just a little assistance on the part of parents. However, rather than engaging Jane in a dialogue about possible solutions, Lilly succumbed to her own anxiety and her desire to lessen Jane's distress by immediately advising Jane to tell the other girls if they did not want to play with her then she did not want to play with them.

While one can debate whether Lilly's suggestion would prove helpful to Jane in dealing with her peers, the consequence of Lilly quickly telling Jane what to do and not involving her in considering other possible solutions deprived her daughter of an opportunity to strengthen her problem-solving skills.

We believe that a more productive response would have been for Lilly to empathize with Jane's distress and once having done that to engage in a problem-solving discussion. Lilly might have said, "Jane, I can see how upset you are. It certainly sounds as if your friends did not treat you very nicely, especially by not letting you sit at the same lunch table with them. I'd like to hear more, if you have an idea of what might have occurred before lunch. Then maybe we can think about a few ways to respond to them and what way might turn out to be the best." One cannot predict what the outcome of such a comment will be, but from our perspective it strengthens problem-solving skills as well as a feeling of personal control.

Select what seems to be the best option and put it into action. But prepare for what will happen if the best option proves unsuccessful. This part of the problem-solving sequence involves two parts. The first part is straightforward. After carefully considering different solutions, select the one that seems most likely to succeed.

The second part is also equally important. As we all know, what may initially seem to be the best course of action may prove not to be. This is why considering obstacles is so important even as you think through possible solutions. Early in our careers, we learned that what appeared to be brilliant strategies derived in our offices were not as brilliant when put into practice. Moreover, we found that when parents or teachers and children attempted strategies that they helped to design and these strategies didn't deliver the anticipated positive results, all parties felt even more defeated and less motivated to attempt other interventions. At times, good solutions fall short because of our failure to identify and appreciate obstacles standing between the problem and a working solution.

Exacerbating this kind of situation is the anger that often ensued. Parents or teachers would sometimes blame the child if a particular strategy didn't work. One teacher reported, "I was willing to change several of my expectations, but this student wasn't willing to cooperate," while a parent lamented, "My son said he would be more responsible at home if I stopped reminding him of what he had to do. Well, I stopped, but he didn't change his behavior. I think he needs a tough love approach."

Thirteen-year-old Warren kept misplacing one or more of the textbooks needed in each class. He decided to abandon his locker and keep all of his books with him in a backpack throughout the seven-class school day. At first consideration, this appeared a workable solution; however, Warren soon discovered that his thirty-eight-pound backpack was just too heavy and cumbersome to carry through the halls. When he turned while walking to class to greet a friend, he accidently bowled over a smaller student and was sent to the Vice-Principal, backpack and all!

Warren's backup plan was to request a second copy of each textbook to be left in class allowing him to leave his textbooks at home. Warren's science teacher liked this idea so much that he instituted this plan for any student who requested it.

As with Warren, a good solution to a potential problem is to prepare people for the possibility of a strategy not working. Many years ago, we wondered what might occur if after determining with patients or consultees (even the graduate students we trained) a particular strategy to implement, we said, "This plan seems very well thought-out, but I think it may be important to consider the question, 'What if it doesn't' work?'"

We reflected upon the danger of introducing such a question, namely the possibility of it being interpreted as a self-fulfilling prophecy for failure. If people were going to be prepared for possible setbacks, it was necessary to convey an additional message, which took the following form:

"If our first strategy doesn't work, let's think about how you might react. And, very importantly, let's think in terms of what we might learn from the setback in selecting another strategy to use. Sometimes the first strategy used may not turn out to be the most effective one."

It may seem paradoxical that in a chapter devoted to Intuitive Optimism, we would propose introducing the theme of possible failure. However, research by Psychologist, Dr. Gabriele Oettingen, Author of *Rethinking Positive Thinking*, suggests otherwise. She has proposed an important model bolstered by research to demonstrate the need to "combine positive thinking with realism." She advocates the importance of identifying not only one's wishes or goals, but also the obstacles that might arise in realizing these goals as well as ways to overcome these obstacles.

Dr. Oettingen's approach, which she describes as *mental contrasting*, contributed to participants in her studies achieving better outcomes compared with those who focused solely on their wishes or dwelt only on possible obstacles. In effect, when people are prepared for setbacks and obstacles, it is easier for them to cope successfully with these barriers and reach their goals.

We saw 12-year-old Becky in therapy because of her overwhelming anxiety. She was a shy, worried girl, and recent family events had added to her anxiety, including her mother being diagnosed with breast cancer and her father temporarily losing his job but soon finding another.

During the first few months of therapy, Becky's level of anxiety lessened as we examined various ways of coping with her worries. She told us at one point that it reassured her when we had discussions about ways of solving problems since it helped her to feel that there were different solutions to the problems she was experiencing.

In one session, Becky came in upset. She learned from two other girls whom she trusted that her supposed best friend Sara was making up negative stories about her, including Becky not being a "loyal" friend. Becky said she believed this was happening and asked us what she should do.

We explained that it was important for Becky to consider what she thought would be the best way to deal with Sara. Becky explained that initially she thought of not saying anything, but lately, she noticed Sara was running "hot and cold" in terms of their relationship. "I just think I have to say something to her, that I have to tell her what I heard and we have to talk about our friendship."

Continuing to reinforce Becky's problem-solving abilities, we wondered, "How do you plan to do this?"

Becky replied that she had two thoughts: One was to send Sara an email, and the other was to talk with her privately. Given Becky's shy demeanor, we were somewhat surprised when Becky decided to talk with Sara directly.

We next considered what Becky might say. Becky acknowledged that she was nervous but described how she planned to tell Sara that several other girls had mentioned that Sara had said some negative things about her and that she wanted to know where "their friendship stood."

We reinforced Becky's plan and then posed a question referencing an obstacle. We asked, "What if Sara denies she ever said anything negative about you?"

Becky responded, "I never thought about that. I think I would feel stuck."

We explained, "The reason we asked that question is that we think it's helpful to consider how we might reply when we're trying to make changes in our lives and things we don't anticipate come up. Sometimes it can throw us off balance."

Becky asked us how she should reply. While we had an answer, we thought it would be more beneficial to jointly consider different options. Eventually, we arrived at a solution. Although the solution was prompted in part by our questions, Becky certainly felt she had participated in the process.

If Sara told Becky that none of what she was told was true, Becky was prepared to say, "I thought you would say that, but I have to be honest, I believe it is true." We next discussed other possible scenarios, including Sara saying she no longer wanted to be Becky's friend.

In fact, Sara did respond by saying what Becky was told wasn't true. Becky replied in the way she had prepared.

Becky told us, "I didn't know what Sara would say after I told her I thought that was what she was going to say. I was surprised when Sara started to cry and apologized and said she wanted to continue to be my friend."

This event turned out to be a pivotal moment in Becky's therapy. She displayed increased confidence in her ability to successfully confront future problems.

Identify strengths or islands of competence. In Chapter 1, we noted our shift from a "deficit" to a "strength-based" approach and a focus on identifying and reinforcing each child's *islands of competence*. Such a shift does not mean minimizing or ignoring problems but rather spotlighting interests and strengths. When children such as Gavin, the "pet monitor" we described in Chapter 1, are encouraged to actively pursue their *islands of competence* and when these islands are honored by parents and other adults, the instinct of Intuitive Optimism is reinforced.

It is for this reason that we always introduce the topic of strengths or *islands of competence* in our clinical work. For instance, in a session with Mia and Joe, whom we discussed earlier in this chapter, we asked about their daughter Madison's strengths. Mia immediately described how much Madison enjoyed drawing, especially animals, adding that she thought her daughter's drawings were very impressive.

Then, she sadly added, "Madison gets a great deal of joy when drawing, but when she begins to feel down about her reading, she also seems to lose interest in drawing. It's as if all of her energy is drained."

In an individual session with Madison, we asked what she enjoyed doing and what she thought she did very well. Madison quickly mentioned she loved to draw pictures. When we inquired what kinds of things she liked to draw, Madison said, "A lot of things, but most of all I love drawing all kinds of animals."

As Madison said this, her entire face seemed to light up, but the joy was short-lived when she corroborated her mother's observation by noting, "But I've been feeling tired and haven't been drawing too much lately."

We asked Madison to bring some of her drawings to our next session. She did and we were impressed with her creativity and talent. She beamed as she went through her scrapbook describing each drawing in detail. Discussions with Mia and Joe as well as Madison's teacher led to an intervention plan rooted in great part in reinforcing and displaying this *island of competence*.

Madison agreed to take an art class at a local museum, during which she received very positive feedback from the instructor. In addition, Madison's teacher at school enlisted her in completing several drawings of animals that became part of a display in the lobby of the school. Madison was also asked to help first graders at her school learn to draw animals.

These interventions were not intended to have Madison ignore her reading struggles, but rather to lessen the pessimistic outlook she possessed associated with dyslexia. They provided her with concrete ways to experience her strengths. A critical dimension of her therapy was to replace what her father referred to as a "victim's" mentality with a mindset filled with hope that included an appreciation of these strengths. Such an appreciation helped Madison to slowly develop the attitude that while reading might always be difficult for her, she was still a very capable girl.

"Provide opportunities to engage in contributory activities." This strategy to reinforce Intuitive Optimism is closely aligned with the instincts of Compassionate Empathy and Genuine Altruism. As you will learn, while each of the seven instincts can be described individually, a single strategy may in fact serve to reinforce more than one of the seven.

In four of our books framed by resilience theory and written for parents, we described what we call contributory activities as a major activity in promoting hope and resilience. Such activities also play a large role in strengthening Intuitive Optimism. Young children appear to come into the world with an inborn need to help. Three-year-old children will eagerly approach their parents while watching them mow the lawn and ask if they can help. The want to help us cook, take care of younger siblings, rake leaves, build things with our tools, and some even want to drive the car or push the lawn mower.

Some parents report that their children have lost this drive by the middle childhood years. While that may be true in the home environment, what parents often fail to observe is the help their children are providing to their peers or to teachers in school. In research we conducted, we found that some of the fondest memories people have of school—experiences that boosted their optimistic outlook and motivation—centered around being asked to help (e.g., "I remember when a teacher asked me to pass out the milk and straws"; "I loved when I helped stack books in the library"; "I will never forget when I was given an opportunity as a senior in high school to tutor a freshman who was having trouble with math").

Contributing to the well-being of others, regardless of one's age, nurtures a sense of purpose and meaning to one's life. It promotes the belief "I can make this world a better place." One study found that at-risk teenagers became more hopeful and less likely to drop out of high school when asked to read to elementary school students. This sense of purpose, of making a positive difference, fuels Intuitive Optimism.

We offered an example of the power of contributory activities (as well as *islands of competence*) with Gavin, the pet monitor, who taught his classmates about animal care. Let's return to Becky for another illustration of this strategy. Earlier, we discussed Becky to illustrate the importance of problem solving. We also mentioned that her anxiety increased when her mother was diagnosed with breast cancer.

The uncertainty of her mother's cancer prognosis, the disruption in household routines given mother's treatment, the fear of losing her mother, and her father's temporary unemployment, all served to intensify anxiety in this already anxious child. In considering different interventions for Becky, we reflected upon personal control and contributory activities as possible therapeutic forces. There are many events over which we have little, if any, control such as Becky's mother developing breast cancer. However, as we noted earlier, we have more control than we realize in terms of our attitude and response to these events.

Becky joined her parents in a "Walk for Breast Cancer Research." All monies raised from the walk were funded to support research to end breast cancer. Becky was very proud of the number of donors who contributed to her walk. Her gains in therapy, including more confidence in her ability to problem solve, were augmented by raising money for breast cancer research.

These seemingly simple experiences had a powerful impact on Becky's mindset. We frequently remind parents and children that we cannot easily change the physical brain despite promises made by some Website gurus, but we are all capable of arriving at new ideas that enrich our lives. It was obvious from our discussions with Becky that the walk for charity fueled her belief that she was doing something constructive; her efforts provided hope for the future. Intuitive Optimism was strengthened.

Try, Try Again

"If at first you don't succeed, try, try again" wrote American educator Thomas Palmer in his *Teacher's Manual* in 1822. To persist requires a mindset willing to try again in the face of challenge, adversity, or mistakes. This does not imply the judgmental quality of "try harder." Rather, the critical component of such a mindset is the intuitive, optimistic belief that perseverance together with the implementation of new problem-solving strategies can lead to success. In light of humankind's history, an appreciation of Intuitive Optimism as a key component of *Tenacity* is easily understood.

Chapter 4
Intrinsic Motivation

Alexa and Dawn are four years of age. They attend different preschool classes. They take great pleasure coloring. It is their favorite free time activity. Their finished products range from stick figures with hands and legs often emanating from a large head as is not unusual for their age to what may appear like scribbles, but are perceived by these two children—as well as their parents—as works of art.

Alexa's teacher thought that the children who delighted in coloring and drawing pictures would enjoy this activity even more if given a tangible reward after completing each picture. She also thought that providing a reward for this activity even to those children who did not appear as interested in drawing would motivate them to pick up crayons and pencils. Dawn's teacher did not think a reward was necessary to enrich the experience of drawing and coloring.

Do you think the introduction of a reward would have any impact on Alexa, her like-minded peers, and all of the children in the class? A frequently cited study published nearly 50 years ago by researchers Drs. Mark Lepper, David Greene, and Richard Nisbett examined these phenomena. They asked what would occur with 3–5-year-old nursery school children when external reinforcers were introduced for a favorite activity. Would such a prize heighten a young child's interest in the activity as Alexa's teacher assumed? Or would it not?

These researchers observed a preschool class and identified those children who chose to draw whenever there was a period of free time. They then divided these children into three groups. The first group they called the "Expected Award" group. They showed each child in this group a "Good Player" certificate featuring a blue ribbon and the child's name. They explained that each child would receive this award when they finished their drawings.

A second group was designated the "Unexpected Award" group. These children were also given the "Good Player" certificates when they finished their drawings, but they were not told in advance that this would happen. The third group was labeled the "No Award" group. These preschoolers were asked if they wanted to draw, but they were neither promised before nor given a certificate after they completed their drawings.

© Springer Nature Switzerland AG 2021
S. Goldstein and R. B. Brooks, *Tenacity in Children*,
https://doi.org/10.1007/978-3-030-65089-6_4

Two weeks later, the teachers of these groups put out paper and markers during the free play period while the researchers secretly observed the children. A central question in this study was whether involvement in one of the three groups two weeks earlier would have an impact on the children's current behavior. If so, what would it be? One prediction was that an award given two weeks earlier would not have any impact on the child's behavior currently. Another possibility, rooted in the tenets of extrinsic motivation or what author Daniel Pink in his book *Drive* labeled "The Motivation 2.0 Operating System," was that those children promised and given a reward for drawing would display even greater interest in engaging in that activity in the future.

These researchers found that in fact even two weeks later, the presentation of an award had an impact on the preschoolers' interest in drawing! However, the findings were not in keeping with what might have been hypothesized by the 2.0 System described by Pink. Children in the "Unexpected Award" and "No Award" groups drew just as much, with the same enthusiasm as they had before the experiment. In contrast, children in the first group—the ones who had expected and then been given an award—displayed much less interest and spent less time drawing currently. Were the children in this group discouraged by being given a promised award for an activity they had previously engaged in for sheer pleasure?

Without suggesting an interpretation that goes far beyond the data, it appears that the awarding of certificates or prizes, a common practice in many classrooms, had seemingly transformed play into work. It is important to point out that it wasn't necessarily the reward that reduced the children's interest since when children didn't expect a reward, receiving one had little impact on their intrinsic motivation. Only what we refer to as *contingent* rewards—if you do this, then you'll get that—had a negative effect. In fact, multiple studies over many years have found that contingent rewards, the foundation of nearly all behavior modification programs, are rarely successful in producing lasting changes in behavior or attitudes. When the rewards stop, children and adults usually return to the way they behaved before the program began. As author Alfie Kohn pointed out in his book *Punished by Rewards* over twenty-five years ago, extrinsic motivators do not alter the emotional or cognitive *commitments* that underlie behavior–at least not in a desirable direction. A child promised a treat for learning or acting responsibly has also been given a reason to stop doing so when there is no longer a reward to be gained.

The results of Drs. Leeper, Greene, Nisbett study invite the question of why extrinsic motivators not only failed to heighten interest in a favored activity but actually decreased interest in that activity. In Chapter 2, we referred to the work of Harvard Psychologist, Dr. Robert White. In 1959, Dr. White posited that there is an inborn need to master one's environment; that we all possess a "drive for effectiveness." This natural drive, fueled by curiosity, interest, and mastery, is thwarted when extrinsic reinforcers are introduced solely in a contingent way. It is as if such reinforcers detract from a sense of enjoyment and mastery.

Self-Determination Theory (SDT), a theory of motivation in keeping with Dr. White's position, has been proposed by Psychologists Drs. Edward Deci and Richard Ryan. They call into question the effectiveness of a contingent reward and punishment model (i.e., extrinsic motivation) as a catalyst to motivate children and adults. Instead, a basic premise of their theory is that people will be intrinsically motivated to engage in tasks in which certain inner needs are being satisfied. In one study, they paid children to read. These were children chosen because they already enjoyed and chose to read on their own. When the payments stopped, many of these children actually stopped reading!

Drs. Deci and Ryan originally identified three needs but then added a fourth after conducting further research. These needs include (1) belonging and connectedness, (2) self-determination and autonomy, (3) competence, and (4) a sense of purpose in one's life. Let's briefly define each of these and then discuss each in depth.

Belonging and connectedness. Belonging is the need to be attached to others as well as to give and receive attention to and from others. Belonging provides children with a sense of safety and security. Belonging begins with family and is a strong and inevitable feeling that exists in human nature. In Chapter 1, we described the concept of charismatic adults, a concept first introduced by the late Psychologist Julius Segal and emphasized in our book *Raising Resilient Children*. Such adults were seen as being connected to and held in a special place in a child's heart and mind no matter the circumstances. Whether it is to family, friends, co-workers, a religion, or anything else, people tend to have an inherent desire to belong, be connected, and be an important part of something greater than themselves. This implies a relationship that is more than a simple acquaintance or familiarity.

Social Psychologists, Drs. Roy Baumeister and Mark Leary posit that belonging-ness is such a fundamental human motivation that we experience severe consequences if we believe we don't belong with someone or somewhere. If it wasn't so funda-mental to our nature, then lack of belonging wouldn't have such dire consequences on any of us. Think of how you have felt when excluded from a desired group or person. Think about how hurt your children appear when they are excluded by desired peers. This desire is so universal that the need to belong is found across all cultures and different types of people.

Self-determination and autonomy. This is the second need. Offering people extrinsic rewards for behavior that is intrinsically motivated undermines self-determination and autonomy as children grow less interested in the activity. In the preschool experiment we just discussed, intrinsically motivated behavior becomes controlled by external rewards, which then undermines a child's sense of autonomy. We can't tell you how many times youth we work with tell us they only need to complete a certain amount of work in a class in order to earn a desired grade. The goal of earning the grade, an extrinsic reinforcer, had replaced the quest for knowl-edge. Dr. Deci and his colleagues in the same series of studies also found that giving people unexpected positive feedback on a task increased their intrinsic motivation to complete the task. Remember how you felt when you brought a successful assign-ment home from school and your parents proudly displayed it on the refrigerator. In fact, giving positive feedback on a task served to not only increase intrinsic motiva-tion but to also decrease extrinsic motivation for the task. Consistent with this view, reserachers, Drs. Robert Vallerand and Greg Reid discovered that negative feedback has the opposite effect (i.e., decreasing intrinsic motivation decreased the drive and interest in developing competence).

Drs. Deci and Ryan shifted away from labeling behavior as either extrinsically or intrinsically motivating. Instead, they recommended that behavior be categorized as either controlled or autonomous. The former was seen as behavior that comes from forces outside oneself, while the latter was seen as behavior rooted in a sense of volition and choice.

Competence. Competence is the third need. It has many different meanings. It is one of the most diffuse terms in the organizational and occupational literature. However, for our purpose, competence can be best described as an ability to understand, successfully perform in, and master our world. If a child possesses confidence that he/she can do those three things when facing life's challenges and opportunities, then they will feel competent. Competence is both a belief and an action. Competent people believe they can sufficiently use their know-how and skills to manage and succeed at the tasks they encounter. We all possess a drive for competence and mastery. It is essential given the many developmental challenges we face and the extraordinary volume of knowledge we must acquire as we grow. The drive for mastery is evident from an early age. Consider the stamina of a very young child who continues to attempt to walk despite falling down many times. And the joy children display when they are able to do so!

Purpose in life. Purpose, the fourth need, is viewed as representing the desire to believe that one's activities enriched the lives of others, that what we do goes far beyond the benefits that come our way. In his book, Daniel Pink observed, "Autonomous people working towards mastery perform at high levels. But those who do so in the service of some greater objective can achieve even more. The most deeply motivated people—not to mention those who are most productive and satisfied—hitch their desires to a cause larger than themselves." The need to feel a sense of purpose is captured in the impact of "contributory activities" that we described in Chapter 3.

Our colleague and educator Mr. Rick Lavoie in his book *The Motivational Breakthrough* also offers a valuable theory of motivational needs. He proposed that there are six primary needs or forces that serve as sources of motivation in all children and adults. He noted that these forces are distributed differently in each of us and that is why certain situations are more intrinsically motivating for some children than others. He labeled them the 6 P's. They include the need for: Praise, Power, Projects, Prestige, Prizes, and People-Oriented.

In Drs. Deci and Ryan, and Mr. Lavoie's models when these needs are fulfilled, intrinsic motivation blossoms. Conversely, when these needs are unmet, intrinsic motivation fails to develop and may even diminish. Drs. Deci and Ryan observed that leaders and managers in too many environments resorted to a reward and punishment approach. They cautioned against the use of contingent reinforcers not only with children but with adults as well. Daniel Pink also wrote, "This is a really big thing in management. When people aren't producing, companies typically resort to rewards or punishment. What they haven't done is the hard work of diagnosing what the problem is. You're trying to run over the problem with a carrot or stick." We agree, but don't unequivocally oppose the use of rewards especially when paired with a conscious effort to build intrinsic motivation.

Daniel Pink summarized the limited conditions under which extrinsic motivation may be beneficial. For Mr. Pink, the emphasis is on the word *limited*. "For routine tasks, which aren't very interesting and don't demand much creative thinking, rewards can provide a small motivational booster shot without harmful side effects. In some ways, that's just common sense."

From our perspective, Intrinsic Motivation as an instinct of *Tenacity* is closely aligned with the models advanced by Drs. Deci and Ryan, and Mr. Lavoie and far apart from the behavioral theory and practice of external rewards and punishments. Viewed as an instinct, intrinsic motivation resonates with the concept of *flow* introduced by Psychologist, Dr. Mihaly Csikszentmihalyi. Dr. Csikszentmihalyi's theory posits that people are happiest and most productive when they are in a *state of flow*—defined as a state of concentration or complete absorption with the current activity or situation.

Dr. Csikszentmihalyi has characterized *flow* as an optimal state of intrinsic motivation. In an online interview with Mr. John Geirland of *Wired* magazine in 1996, he described flow as "being completely involved in an activity for its own sake. The ego falls away. Time flies. Every action, movement, and thought follows inevitably from the previous one, like playing jazz. Your whole being is involved, and you're using your skills to the utmost." Although *flow* as described by Dr. Csikszentmihalyi seems far different from what preschoolers who enjoy drawing experience while engaged in that activity, it may be more alike than we realize. With pencil or crayon in hand, they may be completely involved in an activity for its own sake. And then the enjoyment of that activity is interrupted by an adult offering a prize. Sadly, as we observed in Chapter 2, far too many schools introduce extrinsic reinforcers early in a child's life. In fact, it has been our experience that the more a child struggles with achievement, behavior, and socialization in school, the more extrinsic reinforcers are offered in the form of points, charts, and prizes. We propose instead asking the following question that emanates from the research of Drs. Deci and Ryan:

"What can parents, teachers, and other caregivers do to create home and school environments that satisfy the needs for belonging, self-determination, competence, and purpose?"

More specifically, in terms of *Tenacity*, the question may be posed in the following way: "What can parents, teachers, and other caregivers do to create home and school environments that reinforce the instinct of Intrinsic Motivation?" Let's examine some possibilities.

The Need to Belong and Feel Connected

Relationships and a feeling of connectedness are essential ingredients to shepherd all of the instincts of *Tenacity* toward fruition. Children will be more motivated, excited, and eager to engage in tasks in the presence of adults conveying acceptance, encouragement, and love. In contrast, when negative emotions dominate parent–child relationships, intrinsic motivation is diminished.

Children are more likely to experience a sense of belonging and connectedness in their families when they feel acceptance and unconditional love from their parents. The joy of intrinsic motivation suffers when conditional love dominates a parent–child relationship. Conditional love is fostered when parents mistakenly fail to honor the interests of their children, instead offering contingent reinforcers for almost everything their children do. Many caring parents fall into this trap over and over. In fact, it is seductive. As our children struggle in any area for any reason, we quickly default to contingent rewards often stealing away the child's opportunity to find an intrinsic path to success.

Thirteen-year-old George, a seventh grader, was referred to us because he had set a fire in school. It was what the principal sarcastically called a controlled fire. George took one sheet of paper, lit it on fire with matches he found in the kitchen at home, and tossed the paper into an empty wastepaper basket. Although the act of lighting a fire was not to be minimized, the principal assumed that the manner in which George lit the fire indicated he was not attempting to burn down the school. However, the principal added, "But something worrisome is going on."

George was described as a shy, young adolescent with few friends completing minimal passing work in school. He struggled with a reading disability as well as fine and gross motor challenges. His struggle to read and write effectively was now adversely impacting him in nearly every middle school class. In sharp contrast, George's 16-year-old sister, Linda, displayed excellent interpersonal skills, was a star athlete and an A student. Their parents, Missy and Max White, recounted their own childhoods as similar to that of Linda, characterized my many friendships, and success in sports and academics. Their achievements followed them into their adult lives.

During our first meeting with Missy and Max, they immediately voiced how disappointed they were with George and how proud they were of Linda. While acknowledging George's documented learning problems, they still offered a common, though incorrect opinion, "If George wanted to, he could turn his life around. He's lazy and always has been. He never assumes responsibility."

They described that they and the school had often resorted to using a point system to motivate George to complete school work and meet family responsibilities, but after an initial burst of activity, neither positive nor for that matter negative consequences (no online gaming with friends) appeared to alter George's behavior.

As is our practice, we asked the Whites what they felt George did well, specifically wondering when were the occasions they witnessed their son most motivated and engaged in any task.

Missy and Max glanced at each other with an uncomfortable look. Max replied, "We're somewhat embarrassed to tell you. We just don't think it's the kind of activity that a 13-year-old boy would be spending much of his time doing." The manner in which Max said this seemed to imply that he was referring to some kind of antisocial behavior. Fortunately, this was not the case.

His reluctance to identify George's interests and *island of competence* captured the disconnect Missy and Max felt with their son, a feeling George confirmed in an individual therapy session with us. Finally, Max answered our question. "George likes to garden and take care of plants. That would by okay if he did well in school and was involved in other activities. We tried to restrict his activities in the garden unless he finished his homework but that too soon failed. How can a 13-year-old be so interested in plants?"

This disconnect was further illustrated when we asked the Whites to tell us about one of the most positive moments they can remember having with their son. We thought it was very revealing that eventually each of them recalled a time before George had started kindergarten. Missy teared up as she reported, "I remember when George was about four or five, he loved when I read him bedtime stories. His favorite was *Goodnight Moon*. As I read to him in bed, he would snuggle up to me."

Missy wiped away her tears. Before we could inquire about what prompted her crying she said, "It's very emotional for me to talk about those times with George. I felt so close to him then, but we've grown further and further apart. I don't think he even likes to be with Max and me anymore."

We empathized with Missy and inquired when she started to feel this emotional detachment from George.

"It seemed to take place over a few years, but I know it became greater when homework came into the picture and when George showed little interest in playing any team sports like T-ball or soccer. I remember when he was about seven years old, Max and I offered him some kind of prize if he played soccer. We basically forced him into playing. It was painful to go to his games and watch him. He struggled to run. He was so uncoordinated that he could barely kick the ball. By the second game he seemed so disinterested while the other kids seemed to be having so much fun."

Max nodded as his wife said this and then added, "It was so much easier with Linda. It was a joy to go to her games. We didn't have to offer her a reward to play soccer or any sports. She just loved doing it."

We asked, "Like you mentioned George loves to garden and take care of plants?"

Missy replied, "I never thought about it in quite that way, but I would say that's true." And then in one of those ah-ha moments we've experienced with parents in consultation, Missy observed with tears swelling up again, "But we haven't supported or really shown an interest in the things that George loves to do in the same way we've supported the things that Linda loves to do."

Max listened closely to his wife's remarks and observed, "But it was easier to support the things that Linda did. They were things we loved to do as kids and even as adults. And as I mentioned before, she always seems so involved with her activities."

In our subsequent sessions with the Whites, we encouraged them to reflect upon their unrealistic expectations for George as well as their frustration and anger that he was not living up to these expectations. Slowly, they formulated more realistic goals and, very importantly, began to view George's interests as strengths rather than as some kind of pathology not befitting a 13-year-old boy.

This shift in mindset served as a catalyst for their supporting George's participation in a horticultural show, which they attended. Max told us, "I can't recall the last time I saw George so excited and motivated. He spent hours potting a group of cacti and was so animated when telling people at the show about what he had created."

Instead of using George's *island of competence* of gardening as a reward to motivate him to do his schoolwork, the Whites created non-contingent opportunities for George to expand and develop his intrinsic motivation in an activity that brought him joy. As the Whites began to honor and encourage the expression of George's passions, as they developed more realistic expectations for him and stopped comparing him with Linda, their connection with their son slowly grew. They recognized that his learning problems and his lack of interest in sports did not define him. He possessed other qualities and abilities that were worthy of their attention.

After our consultation with George's educators, the Principal invited him to plant some flowers near the school's entrance. Each day as he entered the building, he was greeted by the flowers he had planted. He also brought plants for the front office of the school, even an Orchid he had grown for the Principal. A sense of belonging and connectedness had been established. The Principal also asked George to start a Grounds and Garden Committee to advise and assist the school custodian take care of the flower beds around the school. Similar to Gavin, the boy we met in Chapter 1 who became the pet monitor, George's strengths were displayed in the school setting. As a result, his intrinsic motivation to confront rather than flee from academic challenges increased as he became increasingly comfortable in the school environment.

In research, we conducted that involved students of all ages answering the question, "What can an adult in the school say and do on a regular basis that helps you feel you belong and are welcome in the school?" we learned that two of the most frequent answers were "greet me by name" and "smile." George's teachers and other staff made an increased effort to greet him with a warm smile and to comment on his flowers and plants.

The Need for Self-determination and Autonomy

In our workshops, we often ask parents and professionals the following question, "Who likes to be told exactly what to do and have no say in anything that they do?" Often this question is met with smiles, which we even exaggerate further by proclaiming, "If any of you answer that question in the affirmative, we will arrange for intensive therapy."

Intrinsic Motivation flourishes when we believe that our voice is being heard and respected and that we have input into situations that impact on our lives. When the strengthening of this instinct is discouraged by parents and other caregivers, it is not surprising to see frustration, anger, and a seeming lack of motivation become dominant forces in a child's life. Gallup polls of students as well as adults in the workforce indicate that those who are labeled as "disengaged" often report that they believe that they have little, if any, say in the school or work environment.

What is it that parents can do to reinforce the instinct of Intrinsic Motivation in their children? Even when children are just toddlers, we can provide choices for them to make. The younger the child, the fewer (two is often enough) and simpler the choices to make. Here are several examples that we would guess are familiar to you:

"Do you want to play with this game or this game?"

"Do you want to put your toys away in this box or that box?"

"Do you want to wear the yellow shirt or the red shirt?"

"Do you want me to remind you 5 or 10 minutes before it's time to go to bed?" (You can even use a timer.)

"Would you like to play your favorite game on the computer for 10 or 15 minutes?" (Most, if not all, children will select 15 minutes, but they are more likely to adhere to the 15-minute limit since they made the choice.)

Some may question if these kinds of simple choices will have a noticeable impact on the reinforcement of intrinsic motivation. We believe that each choice a child is offered serves to strengthen a sense of personal control, a dynamic we discussed in Chapter 3. We should note that the power of having choice is not confined to early childhood. Genuine choices fortify intrinsic motivation at any age and in any setting.

As children develop emotional and behavioral regulation, and critical thinking to guide behavior, simple choices offered by parents can be extended to inviting their participation in more complex family decisions. We are not suggesting that parents abdicate their responsibilities; rather that they allow their children and teenagers to assume increasing input into matters that pertain to their lives. When parents micromanage their children's activities, when children and teens feel that their parents are arbitrarily dictating what is to be done, intrinsic motivation will become a lost commodity.

If Intrinsic Motivation is understood as an inborn instinct driving each of us to seek fulfillment, children will react negatively when expression of that instinct is frustrated. They may refuse to engage in certain activities, even should parents offer rewards as Missy and Max attempted to do to prod George to play soccer. Or, especially once they reach their teen years, they may resort to behaviors that are self-defeating and/or dangerous such as drug use or a refusal to do schoolwork in order to prove there are areas of their lives that they control.

To help parents assess the degree to which they are supporting their children's self-determination and intrinsic motivation, we request that they consider the following questions:

"If we were to interview your children and ask them what choices or decisions they would like to make about their own lives but are not allowed to do so, what might they say?"

"If we were to interview your children and ask them what choices or decisions they make about their own lives, what would they say?"

"What are one or two decisions your children have made that pertain to their lives that you have supported in the past few weeks?"

When we posed these questions for consideration at a parents' workshop, a partic-ipant said, "If we give our 15-year-old daughter an inch, she wants to take a mile." We asked him to elaborate.

"We negotiated that when she finished her homework, she could spend a half-hour on one of those Aps kids use to talk to all of your friends. She wanted 45 minutes, but we told her that a half-hour was the limit. She's very sociable and she could stay on for two hours if we didn't set limits. But she constantly tests limits. She's rather strong-willed."

His wife agreed with what he said.

We asked if their daughter was meeting her other responsibilities as well as getting enough sleep. Interestingly, they answered in the affirmative. They also noted that they knew and liked the friends with whom she was speaking. Since their daughter was meeting her other commitments and was not going to bed very late, we wondered what their reservation was to go from 30 to 45 minutes with her friends.

The woman answered, "My husband and I thought 30 minutes was a fair limit."

We looked at her husband and said, "Earlier you used the word 'negotiated.' What did you mean by that word? Do you think your daughter saw it as a negotiation?"

He smiled and said, "To be honest, I don't know if it was a negotiation. We told her once she finished her homework she could have 30 minutes of time with her friends."

We observed, "Since your daughter seems to be meeting all of her responsibili-ties, what do you think would happen if you told her that you realize she is being responsible and that you feel it would be okay for her to have 45 minutes of time?"

The wife replied, "The problem is that knowing my daughter she is likely to go over the 45-minute limit. And then if we interrupted her to tell her time is up, she would say we're inflexible and don't give her any room. What should we do then?"

"That's a good question. We can suggest one possible strategy that continues to reinforce your daughter having some input and ownership for decisions in her life but also provides you with a safety net should she go beyond 45 minutes."

The husband jumped in and said, "Please tell us."

"It's a strategy that other families with whom we've worked have used success-fully. You can tell your daughter that you're confident that she will adhere to the 45 minutes, but sometimes people can get so involved talking on the phone that they lose track of the time. You can add that since you don't want her to think you're nagging her if you remind her that the 45 minutes are up, you would like her to tell you how she would want to be reminded of the time without her thinking you're nagging her."

We then shared the story of a teenage boy who initially thought he was being funny when he asked his parents to hold up a sign to remind him to complete a task, but it worked out very well. Since it was his idea that they hold up a sign, it was difficult for him to say they were nagging him when they did so. We emphasized that a key goal of this kind of strategy was for a child or adolescent to gain a sense of ownership, which would reinforce his or her intrinsic motivation.

These parents said it was an interesting way of approaching the issue and they would attempt it. A few days later, they contacted us to report that their daughter "bought into" the idea of a reminder; she requested that the reminder comes in the form of a text. Not surprisingly she was pleased to be given the 45 minutes with the additional stipulation that any time on her phone could not go beyond 9:45. Although the strategy had only been in place for a few days, thus far they did not have to use reminders since their daughter monitored the time herself.

The Need to Feel Competent

This particular component resonates with our focus on strengths. In Chapters 1 and 2, we detailed our shift from a *deficit* to a *strength-based* approach that entailed identifying and reinforcing each child's *islands of competence*. As illustrations, we reported Gavin being appointed pet monitor of his school and Madison, who was struggling with reading, being engaged in drawing, an activity that brought her satisfaction and admiration.

Earlier in this chapter, we wrote of George and his passion for gardening. Given his learning problems and his difficulties with fine and gross motor movement, he showed little interest in academics or sports but was highly motivated when involved with gardening. When George's parents eventually encouraged the expression of his *island of competence*, their relationship with their son improved, especially as he sensed their acceptance. Relatedly, his comfort in school was heightened when his strengths were displayed in that venue as well.

Intrinsic Motivation will be dampened when children are required to engage in tasks that they perceive as highlighting their weaknesses. In such a situation, their main motivation will be to escape from such tasks. Recall Gavin's comment, "I used to think it was better to hit another kid and be sent to the principal's office or hide behind the bushes than be in the classroom where I felt like a dummy."

Some psychologists have labeled such behavior an expression of "avoidance motivation." This raises an interesting question. If as Dr. Robert White suggested there is an inborn drive to master one's environment and if as we propose Intrinsic Motivation is an instinct, why would this inborn drive or instinct be hijacked and transformed into avoidance. We raised a similar question about Intuitive Optimism, and in subsequent chapters, the same question can be posed for all of the seven instincts—namely, what derails them from reaching fruition?

In terms of avoidance motivation, we posit that children (and adults) will avoid tasks that they perceive as insurmountable—tasks that will eventually end in failure and humiliation as well as in physical and emotional fatigue. We are certain that at some point in our lives all of us have resorted to avoidance motivation, but typically the avoidance has not prevented us from moving forward in major areas of our lives. However, that is not the situation for some children. They believe that they have few, if any, *islands of competence* to counter their weaknesses and failures so that avoidance motivation becomes a pervasive force in their lives. Almost all their energy and attention are directed toward an escape mode.

We are more likely to engage in tasks that display our competencies. When *islands of competence* are displayed, even within what we call a "self-perceived ocean of inadequacy," their emergence has a ripple effect. In our experience when children such as Gavin, Madison, and George are recognized for their strengths, they are more willing to venture out and build upon other challenges that have proven problematic. Avoidance of challenges is replaced by a willingness to confront adversity with increased confidence and motivation. Success on one *island* leads to success in other areas of one's life.

It is also equally important to consider the attributions or inferences children make about the causes of their successes and failures. In a series of studies with elementary students, Educational Psychologist, Dr. Dale Schunk and colleagues found that third-grade children who were praised over several sessions for their ability (i.e., "You're good at this.") showed greater skill acquisition and self-efficacy than children praised for their effort (i.e., "You've been working hard."). As with any research, others including Dr. Carol Dweck, emphasize the importance of praising effort along with ability. In another series of studies, the pairing of extrinsic reinforcement with efforts at developing intrinsic motivation for good behavior led to the expected improvement. But unlike extrinsic reinforcement only studies, when the extrinsic reinforcement was stopped, good behavior continued. The lesson we learn is that even contingent reward can have lasting positive effect, but it must be paired with the development of and belief in, intrinsic motivation. Children must believe that it is their effort and ability that leads to change and not only the promise of a reward. The reward is just an extra benefit.

One final thought about the benefits and liabilities of praise. Understanding the forces that guide and shape our children's behavior is more complicated than it appears. In an excellent review of the effects of praise on intrinsic motivation, Developmental Psychologists Jennifer Henderlong and Mark Leeper in 2002 pointed out that because adults rely on praise to both influence children's behavior and to express approval, it is important that its motivational consequences are understood. They wrote: "Provided that praise is perceived as sincere, it is particularly beneficial to motivation when it encourages performance attributions to controllable causes, promotes autonomy, enhances competence without an overreliance on social comparisons, and conveys attainable standards and expectations." In effect, the authors advocated that praise could be effective when used in the service of promoting Intrinsic Motivation.

The Need for Purpose

This need parallels what we referred to in Chapter 3 as contributory activities and aligns closely with the instinct of Genuine Altruism that we discuss in greater detail later in Chapter 7. As we noted, we believe that children possess an inborn need to help. Intrinsic motivation is reinforced for those activities that convey the message, "You are enriching the lives of others."

This message is present at all times in our lives. It is displayed in the faces of four-year-olds when instead of being asked to do their chores are asked to "help out." It is displayed when high school students ready to drop out of school are asked to read a few hours a week to elementary school children. Their motivation to leave school is replaced by the intrinsic motivation to be successful in school. As one student asserted, "How can I drop out? I have younger students depending on me."

This same dynamic is demonstrated when senior citizens volunteer their time to go into schools to read to children or engage in other acts of caring. The universal power of purpose has been highlighted by numerous luminaries including:

"No one has ever become poor by giving. (Anne Frank)"
"No one is useless in this world who lightens the burdens of others. (Charles Dickens)"
"Doing nothing for others is the undoing of ourselves. (Horace Mann)"

We have illustrated the benefits of contributory activities such as Gavin teaching his classmates about taking care of pets, or Becky raising money for breast cancer research, a condition with which her mother was diagnosed. Providing children with opportunities to help others is one of the first strategies we suggest for nurturing Intrinsic Motivation and resilience in children. Parents and teachers enlisting children to raise monies for specified charities have witnessed the strength of commitment and motivation children display when engaged in these endeavors. Have you experienced the enthusiasm of children selling Girl Scout Cookies or raising money for an organization in school? Their requests are difficult to turn down!

Peter, a 10-year-old, diagnosed with Attention Deficit Hyperactivity Disorder (ADHD), was not very happy in school. He readily told us that the most common remark he heard from teachers was to "sit still" and "concentrate," both difficult for him to do for long periods of time, even taking the medication prescribed by his pediatrician. Peter explained that his pediatrician told him the medicine would help him succeed at school. Since he was taking the medicine but still having problems, he wondered if his brain was "in worse shape" than he originally assumed. However, as we have learned in working with children with ADHD, pills do not substitute for skills. The medicine is not a panacea solving every problem one hundred percent. In fact, Peter was now so worried that he would forget a book or an assignment that similar to 13-year-old Warren whom we described in Chapter 3, he never left home or school without all of his books and papers stored in his bulging book bag. Unfortunately, they were thrown totally disorganized into his bag making it difficult for him to locate almost anything, including his assignments.

In one of our sessions with Peter, he brought in his book bag in the hopes we could help him become better organized. A stale odor emanated from the bag, and when he unpacked all of his papers and books on our office floor, he discovered a decaying sandwich to which he exclaimed, "Oh that's where my lunch was." He actually had no idea how long the lunch had been packed in the book bag.

Also apparent was Peter's sense of hopelessness at ever succeeding in school and his feeling that his teachers believed that he was not motivated to succeed. His parents, Al and Mandy, reported that it was becoming increasingly difficult to get him to school on time in the morning, and that he frequently complained of stomach aches. Mandy said, "He's so unhappy at school. He gets so worked up and anxious about school that it wouldn't surprise me if he really has stomach aches."

During our meeting with Peter's teachers, we knew one of our first goals must be to change their mindset from "Peter could stay seated and focused if he tried harder" or "Peter needs more medication" to "Peter wants to succeed in school, but he is feeling overwhelmed." We posed a question we frequently ask in our school consultations, namely, "What is it that we can do differently to help Peter succeed?" In raising this question, we are always careful not to suggest to teachers and/or parents that they have done anything wrong but rather to encourage them to explore new strategies.

We facilitated the discussion by asking Peter's parents and teachers what they viewed as his strengths and what does he do that brings him his greatest enjoyment. Al and Mandy talked about Peter loving to play his favorite video game. Al added, "Although Peter can be quite unfocused, he is much more focused when he shows a couple of younger neighborhood kids how to play the game. It's like he knows he has to slow down and be patient." Mandy added that Peter likes to cook with her and seems very attentive when following her instructions.

These examples reflected what we often find in children with ADHD, namely, they were better able to focus and maintain attention when engaged in tasks that were of high interest, as if the experience of *flow* had been triggered. At the school meeting, we brainstormed how best to translate this information into a realistic strategy so that school would become a more comfortable setting for Peter.

The plan that was devised was to tell Peter that some first graders had difficulty packing up at the end of the day, which was true, and that it would be very helpful if he would be willing to go down to the first-grade class 10–15 minutes before school ended to help them with this task. It would also require Peter to receive some "training" from the school psychologist in packing his own book bag so that he would be more knowledgeable in assisting the first graders.

It was heartening at the end of the meeting to view everyone enthused by this plan. One can never guarantee a plan's success. Consequently, we said that if this plan was not as successful as we would wish, rather than becoming discouraged, we would focus on what we learned from this first attempt when developing a new strategy. In Peter's case, a backup or second strategy was not necessary. Peter quickly jumped at the opportunity to be a "helper" and to receive "training" from the school psychologist. In addition, teachers made certain that they refrained from making comments that could be perceived by Peter as judgmental and implying that he could improve if he just wanted to do so.

A few days after the school meeting Mandy reported that she had not seen Peter so motivated to go to school in years. "He just seems much happier now and can't wait to tell Al and me about the kids he's helping. And his own bookbag, though far from perfect, is much neater than it has ever been."

The Qualities with Which We Are Born

Famed Author, Lecturer, and Management Consultant W. Edwards Deming captured our perspective about motivation when he asserted, "People are born with intrinsic motivation, self-esteem, dignity, curiosity to learn, joy in learning." In our view, being "born with" any instinct is but the first step in nurturing its development to build and strengthen a capable human being. It is our responsibility as parents and caregivers to ensure that these inborn qualities are shaped and reinforced in our children. An accomplished, meaningful life will be the end result of these efforts.

Chapter 5
Compassionate Empathy

Louis was adopted by Charlie and Anita Grace at 4 years of age. His biological parents had their parental rights revoked after many years of neglect and numerous failed efforts to comply with a parenting program in order to have their son returned. In the five years since his adoption, we had completed a number of neuropsychological evaluations with Louis, consulted with Louis's school team, worked with his parents and met with Louis in counseling. Louis was taking three different classes of psychiatric medications. Despite everyone's efforts, Louis continued to struggle, and in fact, his struggles were increasing as he approached adolescence. He was impulsive, demonstrated a low emotional threshold and an intense anger when upset, and displayed little empathy and compassion even when not upset.

Louis had a very difficult time accepting any idea or opinion that was not his. He did not suffer from Autism as we determined that he was capable of understanding and taking another person's perspective. He just did not appear to care. As he told his parents multiple times, "I don't care what you think or feel." Louis demonstrated that belief time and time again with his family, schoolmates, and even pets.

When we discussed empathy and compassion with the Graces, Charlie sadly commented, "I don't think Louis has any compassion. Maybe he did when he first came into the world, but the neglect he experienced taught him not to care about anything or anyone except him. I worry that he will never change."

Despite our best efforts as parents, some children come into the world or suffer early adverse experiences leading to a limited capability to develop and display Compassionate Empathy toward people or animals. Although many experts report that a child's violence against other children or animals often represents displaced hostility and aggression stemming from neglect or abuse, we believe more importantly that these adverse experiences rob children of the opportunity to develop Compassionate Empathy.

Even with many years of therapeutic interventions during his teen years, including a stay at a psychiatric hospital and a residential treatment program, his progress toward incorporating and displaying Compassionate Empathy was limited. As

© Springer Nature Switzerland AG 2021
S. Goldstein and R. B. Brooks, *Tenacity in Children*,
https://doi.org/10.1007/978-3-030-65089-6_5

Charlie observed, the early years of extreme neglect and a lack of attachment to his adoptive parents despite their attempts to be supportive and loving had taken a toll on Louis, a toll that could not be readily remedied.

The Power of Compassionate Empathy

Although scientists have proposed different theories for the concepts of empathy and compassion as well as suggesting ways in which they are distinguished from each other, most define empathy as understanding the world of another person both on an affective and emotional level. In contrast, compassion is seen as drawing upon that understanding in an attempt to improve the lives of others. Taken together, we believe that the concept of Compassionate Empathy is a powerful instinct, one that is implicated in the survival and development of our species.

James Allworth, Head of Innovation at Cloudfare, a *New York Times* bestselling author, and a graduate of Harvard Business School (HBS) described "the most valuable thing they teach at HBS" in a 2012 article posted by *Harvard Business Review*. What do you think he judged that to be?

Empathy!

He asserted, "These probably aren't words that you were expecting to read in the same sentence—Harvard Business School and empathy, but as I reflect back on my time as a student there, I've begun to realize that more than anything else, this is one of the most valuable things that the school teaches."

In reflecting on his experiences at HBS, Mr. Allworth emphasized that empathy helped "you to step out of your own shoes and put yourself into those of someone else." He noted that this quality is often lacking in business and politics, and that it is an attribute that should be cultivated.

Psychologist, Dr. Daniel Goleman proposed that empathy is a critical component of both emotional intelligence and social intelligence. In his 2002 book *Primal Leadership: Realizing the Power of Emotional Intelligence,* Goleman and co-authors Richard Boyatzis and Annie McKee vividly described the impact of empathy. They wrote:

> Empathy is the fundamental competence of social awareness.... Empathy is the sine qua non of all social effectiveness in working life. Empathic people are superb at recognizing and meeting the needs of clients, customers, or subordinates. They seem approachable, wanting to hear what people have to say. They listen carefully, picking up what people are truly concerned about and they respond on the mark.

In our previous writings, we have emphasized the impact that empathy has in determining the quality of our interactions, including the parent–child relationship. It's of interest that Allworth spoke of HBS teaching empathy to its graduate students. We have positioned Compassionate Empathy as an instinctual component of *Tenacity*.

One may question if it is an instinct, then why must it be taught? And why must the teaching extend beyond our childhood to the graduate school years? As we have asserted in earlier chapters in this book and wish to emphasize again, we believe that the seeds of all seven instincts are present from birth, but they require the patient input and modeling of parents and other caregivers to reach fruition. As Allworth observed, the development of empathy is an ongoing process that crosses into our adult lives—a process that we posit is an underpinning of the ongoing development of *Tenacity*.

Before proceeding, we want to address two issues. The first involves defining the concepts of "compassionate" and "empathy," examining the ways in which they differ, and the reasons we integrated them into one instinct. The second highlights research that supports the instinctual nature of empathy and compassion and their rudimentary appearance in the very young child and toddler.

Compassion and Empathy: A Powerful Dynamic

This book represents our first attempt to bring together the concepts of empathy and compassion. We believe that merging the two allows us to more fully capture a major instinctual component of *Tenacity*. Psychologist, Dr. Dacher Keltner, founder of the Greater Good Science Center at the University of California, Berkeley, reported in 2012 that researchers of human emotions have defined compassion as "the feeling that arises when you are confronted with another's suffering and feel motivated to relieve that suffering. Compassion is not the same as empathy or altruism, though the concepts are related. While empathy refers more generally to our ability to take the perspective of and feel the emotions of another person, compassion is when those feelings and thoughts include the desire to help."

Paralleling our view that the instincts comprising *Tenacity* may be understood using an evolutionary lens, Dr. Keltner proposed that "compassion is essential to our evolutionary history, it defines who we are as a species, and it serves our greatest needs as individuals—to survive, to connect, and to find our mates in life." Dr. Keltner noted that "our babies are the most vulnerable offspring on the face of the Earth. We became the super caregiving species, to the point where acts of care improve our physical health and lengthen our lives. We are born to be good to each other."

Ms. Sara Schairer, founder of Compassion It, a nonprofit organization developed to inspire compassionate actions and attitudes, offered a perspective similar to that of Dr. Keltner's in a 2017 article. She wrote that empathy is "viscerally feeling what another feels," citing research related to "mirror neurons" and automatically feeling what another person feels. In contrast, she stated that "when you are compassionate you feel the pain of another (empathy) and then you do your best to alleviate the person's suffering from that situation."

Psychologist Dr. Paul Ekman has studied human emotions for decades and noted in 2010 that most researchers "generally define empathy as the ability to sense other people's emotions, coupled with the ability to imagine what someone else might be thinking and hearing." He differentiated between two types of empathy, *affective empathy* that pertains to the emotions we experience in response to the emotions of others, and *cognitive empathy* or perspective taking that refers to one's ability to identify and understand other people's emotions.

Dr. Ekman believes that while empathy does not involve initiating action to help someone in need, it's typically a vital step toward what he calls *compassionate action*. He outlined a taxonomy of compassion, noting that it may be displayed in various ways, including toward family, other people, and on a global level.

Present from Birth

Nascent expressions of empathy and compassion exist from birth. Dr. Ekman observed, "Empathy seems to have deep roots in our brains and bodies. Evidence of elementary forms of empathy have been seen in very young children, in primates, in dogs, and in rats.... Research has uncovered evidence of a genetic basis to empathy, though studies suggest that people can enhance (or restrict) their natural empathic abilities." This view closely parallels the position we have proposed in this book.

Psychologists, Drs. Erin and David Walsh in an article published in 2019 observed, "Thanks to mirror neurons, infants as young as 18 months old often show some responsiveness to other infants in distress. We don't teach babies how to do this; they are born hardwired to map the experiences of others in their brain and bodies."

In a 2005 article Primatologist, Dr. Frans B. M. de Waal concluded "examples of empathy in other animals would suggest a long evolutionary history to this capacity in humans." He also provided examples of the ways in which empathy significantly contributed to compassionate actions. As one illustration, he spoke of soldiers who could have killed captives without negative consequences but decided not to. "In war, restraint can be a form of compassion."

Several researchers described the early manifestations of empathy In a Roots of Empathy Research Symposium held in Toronto in 2018. Dr. Andy Meltzoff, Co-Director of the University of Washington's Institute for Learning and Brain Sciences, discussed empathy and brain development, noting, "The infant as young as 13-months-old begins to attribute emotional traits and personality to others based on emotional signals from an adult."

At the Toronto conference, Dr. Brian Goldman, an emergency room physician, supported Dr. Meltzoff's position, "The human brain is hardwired to be empathetic." He viewed empathy as a component of kindness or compassion, "the quality of being friendly, generous, and considerate."

In the work of these and many other researchers and clinicians, the capacity for empathy and compassion may be understood as fundamental qualities that exist in rudimentary form from birth. In addition, empathy is conceptualized as having both an affective and cognitive component that contribute to our understanding of the world of others, while compassion is perceived of as actions we initiate to convey caring toward these others.

Reinforcing Empathy and Compassion in Very Young Child Children

We have been asked at our parenting workshops, "When can parents begin to nurture empathy or compassion in their child?" Without hesitation we answer, "From the moment a child is born." Sometimes our reply is met with a surprised or even an amused look followed by the comment, "From birth? What can I do from birth?"

There are many things we can do from the time our children are born to reinforce the development of empathy and compassion. Fortunately, these involve activities that most parents do very naturally. At the Roots of Empathy conference, Dr. Meltzoff cited brain research that demonstrated within the first few hours of birth newborns showed imitative learning, already responding to the actions of others. In one study using EEG (a measure of electrical activity in the brain), a baby watched another baby's foot being touched and remarkably the foot area in the observing baby's "somatosensory cortex lit up."

In describing the findings of this research, Dr. Meltzoff concluded, "Nothing could be a closer self-other connection than this and this is the beginning of the neurobiology of imitation. The baby sees another body move and maps it on to their own so they can imitate it. We believe this is the foundational basis for the roots of empathy." In summarizing a series of findings, Dr. Meltzoff observed, "This is evidence that the baby's brain can regulate based on emotions they see, even when those emotions aren't directed at them."

In considering these research findings, parents should be aware that whenever they pick up and tenderly hold and soothe their babies, when they smile and gaze into their baby's eyes and softly speak to them, they are contributing to the reinforcement of Compassionate Empathy. We have been asked if children can be "spoiled" during their first 12–18 months of life. A frequent example is whether babies should be picked up and held when they continue to cry. As one father wondered after he had read an article about that subject in a magazine, "If a baby cries after being in the crib for a while and you pick him up, won't that rob him of learning to deal with uncomfortable feelings?"

We certainly want children to learn to self-soothe, but we feel comfortable asserting that cradling a distressed one-year-old is not likely to lead to that child becoming spoiled and incapable of learning coping skills. In their 2019 article, Drs. Erin and David Walsh captured this viewpoint by asserting, "As caregivers nurture and care for infants, babies make crucial associations between positive human interactions, reward systems, and feelings of calm and safety. Children who feel safe, secure, and loved are eventually more sensitive to others' emotional needs."

Psychiatrist, Dr. David Sack eloquently articulated the view we propose about nurturing Compassionate Empathy from an early age when he expressed in a 2012 essay, "Babies learn empathy when their parents consistently meet their needs. When they are fussy, scared, hungry, or uncomfortable, the responsive parent works to understand their feelings and cues and makes them feel better."

Dr. Sack embraced the two features of Compassionate Empathy we described above when he observed, "Children who know they can count on a parent or caregiver for emotional support and physical affection are more likely to offer help to others."

As Children Move Beyond Infancy and Toddlerhood

The early nurturing of empathy and compassion sets the foundation for the ongoing development of this instinct in children. There are specific actions that parents can take to facilitate this instinct's maturation.

As we highlighted in Chapter 3, parents serve as the first models for their children. To engage in this role effectively, we encourage you to consider the following questions and use them as guideposts in your quest to reinforce Compassionate Empathy in your children:

"What words do I hope my children use to describe me?"

"What do I *intentionally* say and do on a regular basis so my children are likely to use the words to describe me that I hope they would use?"

"What words do I think they would actually use to describe me?"

"If the words I hope they would use are noticeably different from the words they would actually use, what changes must I make to bring the two descriptions closer together?"

In Chapter 3, when discussing the concept of empathic communication, we asked readers to reflect upon the following questions:

"Would I want anyone to say or do to me what I have just said to my child?"

"In anything I say or do what do I hope to accomplish?"

"Am I saying or doing things in a way that would allow my children to listen to what I have to say and learn from me?"

The following questions relate specifically to the concept of compassion:

"What do my children observe me saying and doing on a regular basis that models compassion towards others?"

"What family activities do I engage in with my children that involve displaying compassion and enriching the lives of others?"

Let Us Remember Self-compassion

In reflecting upon these questions, we wish to introduce a concept closely aligned with compassion conveyed toward others, namely, self-compassion. It is a concept that is receiving increased attention in the psychological literature and has special relevance when we ask parents to consider the behaviors they are modeling for their children to promote Compassionate Empathy. Below we describe an example of the influence of a parent's lack of self-compassion on her daughter's emotional development, but first a brief definition of self-compassion is in order.

Dr. Kristin Neff, a psychologist on the faculty at the University of Texas at Austin, is a prominent researcher and author defining and articulating the dimensions of self-compassion. In a 2012 interview, she described self-compassion as "treating yourself with the same type of kind, caring support and understanding that you would show to anyone you cared about." She continued, "In fact, most of us make incredibly harsh, cruel self-judgments that we would never make about a total stranger, let alone someone we cared about."

Dr. Neff identified three core components of self-compassion. First is *self-kindness* or being gentle and understanding with ourselves rather than judgmental. Second is an appreciation of our *common humanity*, in which we accept that we are not alone and that imperfection is a basic part of all of us. Third is *mindfulness,* by which Dr. Neff means we don't ignore or exaggerate our pain but rather recognize that it's okay to experience negative emotions so that we can effectively deal with these emotions.

We witnessed the impact that a parent's limited self-compassion can have on a child when we were contacted by Wendy Lawrence, a single mother of 12-year-old Isabella. In our initial meeting with Wendy, she identified the concerns she had about her daughter. "Isabella lacks confidence, she frequently puts herself down, constantly says things like, 'I'm not smart' or 'I always say stupid things when I'm with other kids' and she always seems sad. I wish she felt better about herself. It's painful for a parent to see her child so unhappy."

Earlier we mentioned that in our clinical practice after parents have described what they are most worried about in terms of their child's behavior and emotional well-being, we typically ask them what they perceive to be their child's interests, passions, and strengths, or their *islands of competence*. Wendy reflected on this question and replied, "I'm not certain." She then looked increasingly distressed and said, "Isn't this terrible? I can't even tell you what Isabella's strengths are."

We empathized with the struggles she was having to identify Isabella's strengths, adding that sometimes parents can become so focused on addressing their child's problems that they lose sight of their child's strengths. We rephrased our question to make it more specific.

"What was Isabella doing the last time you recall seeing her happy?"

Wendy answered, "I hadn't really thought about that. I think the last time I saw her looking content was when she was making small pottery or putting together little gems to make jewelry. I had bought her some kits so that she could do these things." Wendy looked down at her wrist and said, "Isabella made this bracelet I'm wearing." We noted how lovely it was, to which Wendy noted, "I agree, but when I thanked her and told her how pretty it was, she immediately said she wished it would have turned out nicer. I think anytime I've complimented her, she rejects the compliment. It can be so frustrating. Sometimes I wonder if I should even attempt to compliment her."

As the meeting progressed, we posed several of the empathy questions listed above. As we always do, we explained the importance and purpose of seeing the world through the eyes of our children and asked, "What words would you hope Isabella used to describe you?"

Wendy thought briefly and replied, "That's quite an interesting question. I guess one word I hope she would use is that I'm loving and that I'm encouraging, especially when she's feeling down, that I'm there for her."

When asked what she says or does so that Isabella would be likely to use these words, Wendy reflected, "I often tell her that I love her, she still lets me give her hugs, and I often encourage her to try different things, but that can get frustrating."

We wondered, "What do you mean by frustrating?"

"At times Isabella seems to feel that I'm putting too much pressure on her and that she really can't do some of the things I think she can. The other day she said something that hurt, but I think it hurt because there's some truth to it. She said that she thought I was disappointed in her and then she said that I thought I wasn't a very good mother because she often felt unhappy about herself."

We replied, "That's quite a statement. You said there was some truth to what Isabella said. What do you mean?"

"I don't even think it's any one comment I make, but just the hurt and defeated look on my face. I know I get frustrated and disappointed with her and I must admit I think she was right when she said I judge my parenting based on how I perceive Isabella is feeling. But I think many parents would do the same."

Wendy paused and then continued, "I think part of the problem is that when I see Isabella putting herself down or quitting, she reminds me so much of myself, and unfortunately, that part of myself that I don't like. She can be so hard on herself and I often wonder what I could have done to boost her self-esteem. I'm just not certain."

We continued, "We can get into a further discussion about that, but we have another question we want to raise. We had asked you how you would like Isabella to describe you. The question is what words do you think she would actually use to describe you?"

Wendy observed, "These are not easy questions. I wouldn't be surprised if Isabella said that I behave in ways that I tell her not to behave, that I often come across as insecure, that I give up on things, and that I'm afraid to try different things."

Wendy looked at us and added with noticeable emotion, "I'm certainly a great role model, huh?"

We stated, "It's obvious that you've had many challenges in your life, including as a single parent. What we have to figure out with you are ways you might change the way you see and act toward yourself and the ways you respond to different events in your life. From what you've said, Isabella is very aware of how negatively you view yourself, even noticing that you're asking her to change things in herself that she sees in you. We'll talk more about that in a few minutes, but to help with the discussion we have yet another question. A little while ago we wondered what you saw as Isabella's strengths and passions. Now we're asking what would you say are your strengths?"

Wendy seemed surprised by this question and after a few moments replied, "Just like I had difficulty describing Isabella's strengths, I'm struggling to describe mine right now. I realize as we're speaking that I've become so focused on Isabella and my problems that I haven't taken time to think about our strengths. I really need a little time to think about it."

We were impressed with Wendy's willingness to examine her thoughts and feelings, especially in terms of her self-worth and her relationship with Isabella. After our initial session with Wendy, our next session included both Wendy and Isabella. Given what transpired in this second session and the wishes of both mother and daughter, our therapeutic sessions from the start were with the two of them together.

The content of our meetings captured the substantial role that parental modeling and interactions play in the emotional development of children. In their first session together, Wendy described her concerns about Isabella's lack of confidence and low self-esteem. Isabella countered, as Wendy thought she might, that while her mother wanted her to become more self-assured and positive, her mother displayed the very behaviors that she wanted Isabella to change. With great insight Isabella observed, "My mother wants me to be nicer to myself, but I get very upset when I see how my mother treats herself. And I also get very upset since I think I'm growing up with the same kinds of feelings about myself."

Isabella's statement served as a launching pad for the therapeutic interventions that were to follow. We established as treatment goals increasing self-compassion and self-worth in each of them; we discussed ways for them to remind each other when either resorted to a more self-critical outlook and steps they could take to begin to pursue their passions and islands of competence.

We were aware that modifying deeply entrenched negative emotions and scripts in Wendy as well as Isabella could not be accomplished in just a few sessions. We saw them in what they labeled "small" family therapy for approximately 18 months. This mother–daughter treatment paradigm proved very successful. Wendy was committed to making changes in her outlook and behavior, guided, in part, by the questions we posed, including how she would like Isabella to describe her and what she said and did on a regular basis for her daughter to describe her in the way she hoped.

Wendy told us, "Those questions certainly caused me to do a lot of thinking about how I treated myself, how I treated Isabella, and how I came across to her. I didn't like the answers I gave myself to these questions and knew I had to begin to make changes. I'm so glad I did when I see Isabella's improvement and how much better our relationship is."

One illustration of Isabella's improvement reflects our definition of Compassionate Empathy and also involves an expression of one's *islands of competence*. During our first meeting, Wendy had mentioned Isabella's love of pottery and making jewelry. At a later session, they both decided to support a food pantry in their town by initiating a charity drive that included several other families. Isabella raised money by selling pieces of the pottery and jewelry she had made.

Obstacles to Nurturing Compassionate Empathy

Review the questions we posed above related to empathy and compassion. As you do, we encourage you to engage in the following exercise:

Write down your answers to each question.

For the questions that encourage action on your part (e.g., "If the words I hope they would use are noticeably different from the words they would actually use, what changes must I make to bring the two descriptions closer together?"), write down one or two steps you plan to take to address existing problems.

Next, and very importantly, consider the research of Psychologist Dr. Gabriele Oettingen that we discussed in Chapter 3. Dr. Oettingen, author of *Rethinking Positive Thinking,* proposed that in making changes in our lives, it is not only necessary to specify goals and strategies to attain these goals, but as importantly, to identify possible obstacles that might arise as we pursue our goals as well as ways to cope successfully with these obstacles should they appear.

We have long advocated an approach similar to that offered by Dr. Oettingen. In doing so, we have stressed that consideration of possible obstacles and setbacks should not be construed as inviting a self-fulfilling prophesy for failure, a viewpoint that might appear especially in those who are struggling with issues of self-doubt. Such a negative mindset is less likely to prevail as long as any list of possible barriers to success is accompanied with realistic strategies to overcome these barriers. Awareness of the existence of these strategies promotes a sense of personal control—a belief that while we may have little, if any, control over certain obstacles appearing, what we do have control over is our attitude and response to these challenges.

The following are three typical obstacles that we have highlighted in previous writings that interfere with the expression of Compassionate Empathy in ourselves and our children.

Fear for Our Children's Distress. During a parenting consultation, 8-year-old Amanda's mother Sherrie commented that she often felt desperate about and an obligation to deny her daughter's negative opinions. We asked for an example. Sherrie commented, "Last week when Amanda came home from school I asked about her day. In tears she blurted out that no one liked her in her class. She's made statements like this many times before. It makes me worry and very uncomfortable because I know that it's not true. I've seen her with her classmates when I've volunteered in her class. She has friends. I felt badly when she said this, but I knew she was wrong, so I told her. Boy did that backfire! In tears she told me I never listen to her and ran off crying. I felt terrible, but I also knew she was wrong and wanted her to know."

This experience is common to most parents when children's feelings distort their perceptions particularly about school and friends. In many such situations when parents offer their conflicting opinions, children dig in and become argumentative. In the next chapter covering Simultaneous Intelligence, we will explain this phenomenon and offer strategies to improve children's critical thinking ability. We asked Sherrie to consider for a moment that she is our therapist. Imagine, we commented, if we said to you we were lonely and depressed and you responded that we had no reason to be depressed or lonely and that there were many people in the world far worse off! We probably wouldn't come back for a second visit and maybe even post a review that you were a poor therapist who didn't listen!

Sherrie smiled, "I guess I never thought of it that way. So, you're saying Amanda just wants me to listen. She wants to be heard?"

We agreed and commented, "A good strategy is to Listen, Learn, Empathize and then through compassion offer help if requested. But for certain don't try to talk your daughter out of her feelings, beliefs, and ideas when she comes to you or responds to your questions."

"What should I say?"

We responded. "First take a deep breath before you respond. As parents our immediate response when our children are in pain is to answer in a way to minimize the child's suffering. We suggest you validate Amanda's observation by accepting that what she says is a truthful reflection of her feelings. You might say: 'I can see how much this upsets you, how can I help?' At that moment Amanda may respond that you cannot help. But at least she knows you've heard her. At a later point you might ask again if you can help."

The Baggage We Carry from Our Past. We have often heard parents lament, "I promised I would never say that to my own children since I really disliked it when my parents said it to me. So, I can't understand why I say those things to my own kids." As we witnessed with Wendy, the experiences we bring from our childhood color the ways in which we perceive and react to our children. If we grow up in a home in which our parents displayed little empathy or compassion, particularly at a young age as Louis Grace experienced, it becomes more difficult for us to develop these attributes and apply them in our childhood as well as when we become parents. If our parents don't model these positive qualities, hopefully they will be established by our interactions with other significant adults in our lives who are empathic, encouraging, and compassionate.

Vicky and Arthur Taunton contacted us about their 10-year-old son Barry. Vicky immediately described how Barry never listened to her, that he constantly provoked his 12-year-old sister Chloe and then claimed Chloe started the argument. Vicky asserted, "Barry can drive you crazy, he never takes responsibility for anything he does, he always blames others." Arthur, while attempting to support his wife, offered a different perspective. He felt Barry wasn't as oppositional as his wife described, adding that Vicky was quick to criticize Barry, while always siding with Chloe.

Arthur's assessment triggered Vicky's anger. "I feel that I have to assume the role of the disciplinarian, the *bad parent* in the family because Arthur won't. It may seem like I'm siding with Chloe, but that's because she doesn't act in the negative ways that Barry does. It's easier to be with her. She's more cooperative."

Arthur replied in an empathic way as he looked at his wife. "I know you feel that way and that things have not gone smoothly between you and Barry, but I think you often seem much more understanding of Chloe. There have been times that it's obvious Chloe has provoked Barry, but you yell at Barry and tell him to stop."

Vicky replied, "But I think it's obvious that Barry is the one who constantly provokes Chloe and me."

As the conversation continued, we posed a question we often ask parents, who, if anyone, Barry most reminded them of. We explained that in our experience parents often respond to their kids based on the ways in which they resemble another person in their lives. Vicky and Arthur were intrigued by the question but were unable to offer an immediate answer. Little could we have predicted the way in which that particular question would serve as a turning point in our work with both of them.

A couple of weeks later, Vicky reported, "I told Arthur I had an *ah-ha* moment. I couldn't stop thinking about whether Barry reminded me of anyone and then it suddenly dawned on me. It probably should have dawned on me much sooner since it seems so obvious now. It may explain why I've had so many struggles with Barry and not taken time to try and be more empathic and understanding with him."

We said, "That's quite a comment. So, who does Barry remind you of?"

Vicky observed, "My brother Skip who is two years older than I am." She then recounted that although as adults they have a cordial but not overly close relationship, as kids he constantly verbally bullied her playing upon her emotions. "He told me I was fat, that no one liked me, that he wished he had a brother rather than a sister. He really didn't let up and he could be very hurtful. The problem was that I always felt my parents favored him, perhaps because he was a boy. When I came to them for help they would tell me that all siblings fight, that they each fought with their siblings, and that I had to learn not to be so thin-skinned. I felt they always minimized my feelings and that they didn't care about me."

Vicky said this with noticeably strong emotion. She added that what the *ah-ha* experience entailed was that when she witnessed Chloe and Barry fighting, it stirred up many memories of her relationship with Skip and she didn't want Chloe to feel unprotected from Barry as she felt from Skip. "Even though I knew Chloe often instigated their battles, I felt I had to tell Barry to stop what he was doing, just as I wish my parents had told Skip to back off when he was taunting me."

Whatever the reasons for Vicky's parents' lack of response to her distress, she grew up feeling hurt and vulnerable, emotions that were to be reignited when she observed the behaviors of her own children. Vicky's desire to ensure that Chloe feel protected, unlike her own experience as a child, resulted in a diminution of empathy and compassion toward Barry. Until she had her *ah-ha* moment, Vicky was unaware that her behaviors were creating the same negative emotions in Barry that she had experienced in her relationship with her parents. Once she recognized the childhood forces that dominated her own parenting behaviors, she was able to begin to shift the current negative scripts to more positive ones filled with greater compassion and empathy toward her son.

A Misunderstanding of Empathy. In our clinical activities and presentations, we continue to hear parents voice the following opinion: "If I'm too empathic it will interfere with disciplining my kids, they will take advantage of me." We remind parents that their expressions of empathy and compassion should not be interpreted as contributing to an abdication of their responsibility to reinforce self-discipline in their children and of failing to teach them to be accountable and responsible for their behaviors.

We also emphasize that disciplinary practices are best served when they are free of intimidation and humiliation. When parents ask, "How can I discipline my kids in ways that they will learn from me and be open to changing their problematic behaviors rather than resisting what I have to say?" we assert that discipline is most effective in the context of empathy and a positive relationship.

We worked with Thomas Dooley who was struggling with his seven-year-old son Evan. Thomas resorted to spanking Evan's backside in response to the latter's whining when he was not allowed to watch a certain television show or when Thomas would not buy him a desired toy. In attempting to promote Thomas' empathy, we suggested he place himself in his son's shoes. He quickly retorted, "I don't care if Evan wants to watch a certain show or get a certain toy, he has to learn he can't! And he has to learn that if he whines, I'll give him a reason for whining. I'll make certain he learns that way."

Thomas' use of corporal punishment to stop his son's whining did not solve the problem; if anything, it added to the stress and tension in their relationship. In light of Thomas' strong opinions, we recognized that if he were to entertain a different approach with Evan, we had to model empathy in our work with him. We asked him what he hoped that spanking Evan would accomplish? Thomas replied, "To stop whining. I know he's only seven, but when he whines, he seems like he's even younger than that."

Thomas seemed surprised when we responded, "Like yourself, we also think it's helpful for kids to act their actual age, but from everything you've told us, spanking Evan has not changed his behavior, if anything he seems to whine more. If it's okay can we share some thoughts we have about ways of disciplining Evan that might lead to the changes you would like to see and, we might add, improve your relationship with him?"

We believe that joining Thomas in his parenting goals and doing so in a way that was experienced as empathic and nonjudgmental allowed him to consider alternative ways of responding to Evan. As one example, when Evan started to whine when not permitted to watch a particular TV show that was deemed inappropriate for a seven-year-old, Thomas refrained from yelling at his son. Instead, with a calm demeanor, he told Evan, "I know you want to watch the show, but I don't think it's a show for kids. You can keep whining, but it won't change my mind. However, if you want to watch television, there are two other shows you can choose from."

Equipped with a new, more empathic, less harsh approach for interacting with Evan noticeably improved their relationship. To bolster their relationship even further, we encouraged Thomas to engage in a charitable activity with Evan, explaining the reasons why. They selected raising money for Evan's tee ball team by baking and selling cupcakes together at a fundraiser. Thomas reported how mature Evan was during this activity and how delightful it was to be with him.

A Word of Caution and Hope

We recognize that when we are upset, disappointed, or angry, it may seem like a Herculean task to model Compassionate Empathy for our children. As important as empathy and compassion are in enriching our daily lives, they are not always easy to achieve. Adding to our frustration is that once we begin to display these qualities, the challenging situations we face with our children are not likely to be resolved overnight. Changing negative mindsets and behaviors requires patience and time. Nevertheless, our perseverance in minimizing negativity in our outlook and actions can secure important benefits, including enriched relationships with our children that encourage and nurture the development of Compassionate Empathy.

Chapter 6
Simultaneous Intelligence

Nine-year-old Maddie had just completed third grade. The previous year she was diagnosed with Attention Deficit Hyperactivity Disorder and treated with a psychiatric medication by her pediatrician. Although her parents, Jack and Susan, as well as Maddie's teacher agreed that her ability to sit still, stay focused, and concentrate had improved dramatically, Maddie continued to struggle in school. By the end of third grade, Maddie's teacher expressed her concerns to Jack and Susan. Although in the first two grades in school Maddie easily acquired academic knowledge related to reading, math, and writing, she struggled throughout third grade, falling further behind in her acquisition of knowledge and ability to understand and follow instructions.

Not surprisingly, the initial thought of Maddie's education team including her teacher and Special Educator was that if she were just able to concentrate, focus, and complete work more efficiently the difficulties she was experiencing would be significantly reduced. Unfortunately, as the third-grade year progressed, this was not the case. We met with Maddie's parents in the summer between third and fourth grades after they were referred by a local Social Worker. Maddie's pediatrician was concerned that her continued struggles might be the result of anxiety. After an initial meeting with Maddie, the Social Worker suggested they come see us for an evaluation. In our first meeting with Maddie's parents, they described her as a very pleasant, happy child as long as she was not involved with schoolwork. They reported that even as an infant and toddler Maddie was an easy child to raise, although her parents noted that she did not appear to spend much time focusing on any single task. In fact, as a toddler, they often brought a large number of toys with them when they were out in public, often switching between toys to hold Maddie's interest.

Susan and Jack also expressed their concern that as the third-grade school year was progressing Maddie appeared increasingly disinterested in completing schoolwork. Completion of homework, which in previous school years was not a challenge, had become an increasingly conflicted task as well. Maddie often resisted finishing homework, frequently complaining that she did not understand the work. Her parents noted that even after medication was prescribed and Maddie was able to sit for longer

© Springer Nature Switzerland AG 2021
S. Goldstein and R. B. Brooks, *Tenacity in Children*,
https://doi.org/10.1007/978-3-030-65089-6_6

periods of time it often appeared that she could read but not understand or reason through the material she was reading. They expressed concern that this was the case in math as well. Maddie could complete simple computations but struggled with word problems. Away from school, Maddie enjoyed dance and tumbling. She had a number of friends and was a helpful big sister with her two younger siblings. Her parents described Maddie as a "sweet, loving child."

We met with Maddie to conduct a neuropsychological evaluation. One way to appreciate the difference between a psychological, neuropsychological, and educational evaluation is to consider that an educational evaluation focuses specifically on achievement, what a child has learned relative to reading, spelling, writing, and mathematics. A psychological evaluation often focuses solely on determining if a child experiences and meets the diagnostic criteria for a specific mental health or developmental condition such as Attention Deficit Hyperactivity Disorder, anxiety, depression, or a learning disability. A neuropsychological evaluation focuses not so much on diagnoses or scores but seeks to provide an understanding and explanation of the underlying weaknesses that lead to the child's problems. In doing so, neuropsychologists focus on process more than product. The intent is to identify the reasons the child struggles to manage emotions, remain focused, or acquire academic knowledge, and intervene at the process level.

We completed a neuropsychological evaluation with Maddie. In this evaluation, we began by focusing on four kinds of neuropsychological processes: planning, attention, sequencing, and simultaneous ability. We believe that these four abilities are critically important as children progress through school. Our testing revealed that Maddie was able to plan and strategize. She could pay attention to detail and work with information in sequence. All three of these abilities are key components contributing to the success with which children acquire knowledge. However, in contrast to the other three scores, Maddie's simultaneous ability, or capacity to reason abstractly, was measured as significantly below average and well below her other scores. We also found that Maddie demonstrated average language development and memory. She had taken the prescribed medication just prior to the testing. Not unexpectedly she was focused and completed all administered tasks.

Interestingly, when we evaluated Maddie's academic knowledge, we found that her understanding of basic math, word attack or reading decoding, and spelling, were all in the average range. In contrast, Maddie's reading comprehension was measured as well below average. She could read but had a difficult time integrating and understanding what she was reading. This knowledge was needed to answer questions about the material. This was not a language problem but rather reflected a weakness in Simultaneous Intelligence. This pattern was true as well in math. Maddie understood basic math processes at grade level but struggled to apply these processes efficiently when asked to complete story problems.

As we briefly explained in Chapter 2, Simultaneous Intelligence guides our practical understanding of how elements of a problem fit together into a solution. Simultaneous Intelligence is best defined as the ability to see how all the parts fit together when solving problems. It requires reasoning and thinking. Research from around the world has demonstrated that this instinct is not culture or experience bound.

Academic achievement is often best explained by opportunity. Simultaneous Intelligence on the other hand is not defined by culture or social class. The current conceptualization of intelligence as defined in many public schools incorporates not just thinking but also reading and math achievement. It is for this reason that intelligence tests as traditionally used in the schools have been demonstrated as a good predictor of basic academic achievement. These tests have traditionally included measures of vocabulary, information, and comprehension, very clearly dependent upon experience. Unfortunately, this emphasis created a bias leading to an over identification in our schools of minority children or children living in poverty as intellectually handicapped. The limitations of these children are a consequence of their environment, not an indication of their potential. These four neuropsychological abilities have been measured as equally developed in similar aged children living in such diverse environments as the Australian outback, inner city, or affluent suburbia, independent of socioeconomic level.

We met with Susan and Jack to discuss our test results and introduced the concept of Simultaneous Intelligence to them. We find this concept sometimes difficult to understand. In speaking to parents, we begin by offering these two examples:

1. If I provide you with a defined sequence of numbers such as 2, 4, 6, 8, 10; this very predictable sequence requires very limited reasoning or Simultaneous Intelligence. One only needs to know 10 to predict 12. However, if we provide you with this sequence: 1, 3, 6, 10, 15; knowing 15 or even 10 and 15 is insufficient to accurately identify the next number in this sequence. To do so requires Simultaneous Intelligence. That is, simultaneously appreciating the relationship of every number to every next number to understand that the gap between each set of numbers keeps increasing by 1. The next number in this sequence is 21!

2. The second example we offered to Susan and Jack required them to guess an animal name based on the ten facts we provided. We explained that if we presented these ten facts about an animal but you randomly chose three, you may pick an animal that matches the three but does not match all of the remaining seven. Effective Simultaneous Intelligence requires that you take the time to understand, think about, reason through, and integrate all of the information available when faced with solving a problem. Susan and Jack then pointed out that Maddie struggled to gather needed information when writing a book report. She usually chose one or two facts from the book as her report and seemed overwhelmed when asked to include and integrate more information.

We asked them if they had ever played twenty questions with Maddie. In fact, they had. Jack laughed, "If we pick something in the room for her to guess, she always starts by choosing an object. When we tell her that's not it, she just proceeds to list more objects." When we then asked Jack if he had ever offered a different strategy to Maddie, he responded, "In fact I've tried to teach her how to play twenty questions time and time again, but she just doesn't seem to understand, like you just said, how to think simultaneously. She chooses to pick random facts, in this case objects in the room, hoping to guess correctly."

As we continued to explain how we measure Simultaneous Intelligence, Susan and Jack began describing other situations in which Maddie struggled to consider and integrate all of the facts on an assignment as she attempted to answer the questions being asked.

Susan pointed out, "If Maddie has to read and answer questions, she's great if the questions have to do with someone's name, where they lived, or what they did. But if the question asked why, Maddie can never seem to figure it out."

We will return to Maddie shortly.

Why Do We Think?

Georgie, a teen we worked with commented to us one day, "Life would be a lot easier if I was a dog." When we questioned Georgie, he responded, "I know my dog can think, but not very much. Life would be a lot better if we just did things and didn't have to think about them so much." We smiled, but before we could respond, he continued, "But then we would probably get ourselves into a lot of trouble!" How right he is!

Why did we evolve the ability to think simultaneously or critically to solve problems? Does our thinking help us make better decisions? The obvious answer is yes. Simultaneous Intelligence reflects the ability to combine sometimes seemingly unconnected pieces of information into a single group or whole to better understand, interpret, and solve problems. This facilitates the comprehension of the relationships of and between separate variables and their relation to the problem to solve. Simultaneous Intelligence is critical to every aspect of life. In fact, we would argue the more complex a society, the more important and diversified Simultaneous Intelligence must be.

One of the fathers of neuropsychology, Dr. A.R. Luria, first proposed the concept of simultaneous ability as the foundational core of intelligence in his seminal work, *The Working Brain* in 1973, after studying individuals with brain injury. However, in 2017, scientists, Drs. Hugo Mercier and Dan Sperber argued that if Simultaneous Intelligence (also referred to as reasoning) makes us human and is the source of our knowledge, wisdom, and higher functioning why didn't it evolve further in other animals? Also, if it is really beneficial, why doesn't it help all of us make the best decision the majority of the time? Drs. Mercier and Sperber suggest that Simultaneous Intelligence is not solely an ability used to make better decisions or solve problems. It finds an additional use in justifying our beliefs and actions to others, convincing them through steadfast arguments. Reasoning, they argue, "contributes to the effectiveness and reliability of communication by enabling communicators to argue their claim and by enabling addressees to assess these arguments. It thus increases both in quantity and epistemic quality, the information we can share with each other."

Drs. Mercier and Sperber argue that in order for communication to be reliable there must be some way for people to convey the truth of what they say and also judge the truth of what others say to them. Certainly, one mechanism that evolved to allow us to do this successfully is our ability to determine when someone is lying. However judging others' communication isn't as simple as distinguishing between truth and lies. When faced with varying opinions we must have a means of deciding which of any of them to believe and follow. Drs. Mercier and Sperber point out that we use our reasoning capacity, sometimes unsuccessfully, sometimes successfully, to engage in this process. In a strategic manner, this allows us to anticipate other's disagreement with our beliefs, opinions, and actions. This facilitates our ability to create counter arguments against potential disagreement, engaging what is sometimes referred to as motivated reasoning.

So, what allows us to begin the process to be open to accepting another person's point of view rather than continuing to create counter arguments ad infinitum? If we and others just continued with counter arguments how do we ever move forward to a consensus and cooperative action? Empathy, altruism, fairness, and responsibility all play a critical role in the process of compromise. In fact, the need to advance our steadfast belief that our choice or opinion is correct may in part have driven the evolution of these instincts. In such cases, your initial motivation is to convince others to believe whatever it is you are arguing for. Thus, a seven-year-old child engaged in attempting to convince you to allow him or her to delay bedtime begins by offering reasons he or she believes will lead to an extension of bedtime. However, seven-year-olds possess limited emotional regulation and immature reasoning capacity. Thus, their arguments often appear weak and unconvincing to you. Their failure to convince you may then lead to a demonstration of excessive emotion. This process, as described by Drs. Mercier and Sperber, helps us understand why children spend so much time arguing their requests, position, decisions, and activities, even after it is obvious to us that their arguments are "falling on deaf ears."

What better way to make your case and engage in this process, both internally and with others, than with language. Language is the window into the mind points out author Steven Pinker. Homosapiens' development of language is most likely the principal reason we evolved successfully when other Hominid species failed. Neuroscientist Silvia Bunge notes, "It's not just that we humans have language at our disposal, we also have the capacity to compare and integrate several pieces of information in a way that other primates don't."

Can We Teach Children Strategies to Enhance Simultaneous Intelligence?

You might wonder if children can develop Simultaneous Intelligence by themselves. After all, lots of smart people have managed to think logically without formal instruction. However, more defined experiences facilitate the growth of Simultaneous Intelligence. As an example, children having an opportunity to discuss their ideas with others is a good first step. Moreover, studies find that children become more effective learners when we teach them to explain how they solve problems. Research suggests that explicitly teaching children strategies to enhance Simultaneous Intelligence makes them better problem solvers, effective independent learners, and even enhances their creativity. In fact, the best way to foster this type of thinking is to teach and model these strategies. This is precisely why we propose that Simultaneous Intelligence is instinctual. To develop optimally the genes that foster this instinct must be nurtured by experience. Studies find that children of all ages become better problem solvers when we teach them to create categories and classify items, identify relevant information, construct and recognize valid deductive arguments, recognize common reasoning fallacies, and distinguish between evidence and interpretations of evidence.

Some may question if the teaching of such strategies will stifle creativity and reasoning. We don't agree with this idea. Simultaneous Intelligence is about thinking flexibly and keeping an open mind. Scientist Robert DeHaan reasons that effective critical thinking is the key to creative problem solving. In the next paragraphs we will summarize three studies among many that provide convincing scientific evidence of strategic instruction to improve Simultaneous Intelligence.

In 1986, Psychologist, Dr. Richard Herrnstein and his colleagues gave over 400 seventh graders explicit instruction in critical thinking—a program that covered hypothesis testing, basic logic, the evaluation of complex arguments, inventiveness, decision making, and other topics. From our perspective, these strategies define a firm foundation for effective Simultaneous Intelligence. After sixty 45-minute lessons, these children were tested on a variety of tasks. The project was remarkably effective. Compared to students in a control group, the children provided with critical thinking lessons made substantial and statistically significant improvements in language comprehension, inventive thinking, and even IQ scores!

In another experimental study, researchers Dr. Anat Zohar and colleagues tested 678 seventh graders' analytical skills. Then, they randomly assigned some students to receive critical thinking lessons as part of their biology curriculum. Students in the experimental group were explicitly trained to recognize logical fallacies, analyze arguments, test hypotheses, and distinguish between evidence and the interpretation of evidence. Students in a control group were taught biology from the same textbook but received no special coaching in critical thinking. At the end of the program, students were tested again. Students with critical thinking training showed greater improvement in their analytical skills, and not just for biology problems. The children trained in critical thinking also did a better job solving everyday problems.

Finally, researcher and educator Dr. Philip Abrami and colleagues analyzed 117 studies about teaching critical thinking. The teaching approach with the strongest empirical support was *explicit instruction*—i.e., teaching kids specific ways to reason and solve problems. In studies where teachers asked students to solve problems *without* giving them explicit instruction, students experienced little improvement.

Unfortunately, there is no single strategy to nurture and provide children with opportunities to enhance Simultaneous Intelligence. Our role as parents and educators may sometimes be as simple as asking open-ended questions to guide the thinking process. In other cases, we can allow children to experiment and refine their theories about what causes things to happen. Psychologist Gwen Dewar offers some practical tips that we present and expand on:

Start early. Young children might not be ready for lessons in formal logic. But they can be taught to explain how they solved a problem. They can also be taught to evaluate the reasons given by others. One of our favorite humorous interactions occurred many years ago with six-year-old Jeffrey. Jeffrey was extremely bright and very impulsive. In the course of our initial evaluation, we asked Jeffrey what kind of a job he might like to have when he is an adult. The following exchange took place.

"I want to be in the Navy."

"Why would you like to be in the Navy?" we asked.

"Because in the Navy," Jeffrey answered, "You get to sail around on big ships."

We couldn't help but ask, "So what do you do on those big ships?" expecting that Jeffrey would answer something about guns, submarines, or torpedoes.

Instead, without hesitation, Jeffrey responded, "You sail around and eat lunch!"

For Jeffrey, being in the Navy was like being on a vacation cruise! His parents later told us he had been on such a cruise with his family the previous year. Jeffrey's experiences on the cruise ship led him to reason in a limited way what life would be like on all ships, including being in the Navy. During a later visit, we had a conversation with Jeffrey about how the Navy might be the same yet different from a cruise vacation, helping him to apply Simultaneous Intelligence. We again asked Jeffrey why he liked the Navy?

He reminded us without hesitation, "I like big ships."

"Are there different kinds of big ships?", we asked.

"No, they are either big or little, I don't want to go on a little ship."

Before our meeting we checked out a picture book from the library about ships. We began to thumb through the pages with Jeffrey. Not unexpectedly he was very interested. "Look Jeffrey, there many big ships that do *different* jobs."

Our comment caught Jeffrey's attention as he pointed to a large oil tanker. "What job does that one do?" he asked.

What followed was a fifteen-minute discussion about the characteristics and varied purposes of *big ships*.

As we rejoined Jeffrey's mother in our Waiting Room he loudly exclaimed for all to hear, "Mom did you know there are all kinds of big ships and you can eat lunch and sail around on all of them, but they are not all the same!"

Avoid preaching. When we tell children to do things in a certain way, we should provide a reason beyond just "because I said so" or "because I am the parent." Psychologist Adam Grant compiled current research and came to two notable conclusions: Role modeling selflessness teaches children to be selfless but preaching generosity to your kids after your great role-modeling behavior, actually makes them less generous! Our model for effective communication is to: Listen, Learn, Influence. We ask parents and educators to guide their communication with children by asking the following questions of themselves:

"Do my messages convey and teach respect?"

"Am I fostering realistic expectations?"

"Am I modeling Compassionate Empathy?"

"Am I setting limits in ways that help children learn from rather than resent me?"

"Am I listening and validating what children are telling me?"

"Do children know I value their input?"

"Am I helping children accept and learn from mistakes?"

"Am I comfortable acknowledging my mistakes?"

The answers to these questions should be used to guide your discussions with children in all circumstances. As an astute but sarcastic teen once told us, "I wish my mother could listen to herself when she lectures me, but I think her inner ear must not be working."

Encourage children to ask questions. Parents and teachers must foster curiosity in children. If a rationale doesn't make sense to a child, she or he should be encouraged to voice an objection or a challenge. From the time our children could carry on a conversation, we have played *The Really Big Question Game* with them. We asked questions appropriate for our children's age for which there were no agreed upon scientific answers such as: "Where does the Universe end?"; "Why isn't there any air in outer space?"; or "Why do some trees keep their leaves in winter and others do not?" Sometimes we would ask questions that had specific answers such as: "Why is it warmer in some parts of the earth?"; or "Why does paint dry?" No reasonable topics were off limits. No prizes were awarded either. If we were not sure of an answer we looked it up, or now Google it. Recently, during one such game with one of our grandchildren we asked, "Do Eskimos eat ice cream and if so how do they make it?" Our seven-year-old grandchild answered they did eat ice cream and they made it in the snow. Before we could respond he picked up our cell phone and Googled it! "Look Grandpa, here is how they do it." *Googling* has added an entire new dimension to our game!

Ask children to consider alternative explanations and solutions. It's nice to find the correct answer the first time. But many problems yield themselves to more than one solution and first choices are not always effective nor the best. When children consider multiple solutions, they may become more flexible thinkers. In our first book, *Raising Resilient Children*, we proposed that the ability to successfully solve problems is linked to all features of a resilient mindset. When children have difficulty thinking about problems in different ways or from different perspectives they may appear impulsive, uncaring, or rigid in their thoughts and actions. Often, failing to appreciate that these children are doing the best they can in light of their struggles with problem solving, we describe them in negative ways.

There are effective strategies that can be applied when we teach children to solve problems. For example, we always ask for two backup solutions or strategies in case our first choice fails. We ask children to consider not only the potential benefits of their choice but the challenges or liabilities as well. We are no longer surprised when five to eight-year-old children, because they think in black and white terms, find it a challenge to consider anything but the initial solution they offer. This problem impacts older youth as well. Billy was a very impulsive thirteen-year-old teenager we worked with many years ago. He dutifully followed our strategy to always have two back up plans before you begin with the chosen plan you think is best. Unfortunately, for Billy his challenges with impulse control led him to make the choice he thought best, absent much time thinking. The following incident illustrates this point. Billy explained that his soccer ball was accidently kicked on the roof and though this had happened before and the ball usually rolled off, this time the ball stopped in the rain gutter.

Billy explained: "So, I thought of three ways to get the ball down. I could get a ladder, but we don't have a ladder. I could try to stand on my brother's shoulders but he's not very strong. I could get the key to our motor home parked in the driveway, start the engine and very slowly drive closer to the side of the house. Then I could climb the ladder on the side of the motor home and get the ball. That's the strategy I picked because I knew where the key was hanging in the hall closet."

Before we could respond Billy continued, "I really thought about it. I know how Dad backs the motor home out of the driveway and I really thought I could do it."

We soon learned that Billy had indeed moved the motor home but too close to the house, crushing the rain gutter and creating an even bigger problem! This event led to a discussion with Billy about ways to consider the various potential costs and challenges of different solutions.

Help children to clarify meaning. Children should practice putting their ideas and experiences into their own words while keeping the meaning intact. They should be encouraged to provide explanations and make meaningful distinctions between the reasons for their choices. To help children develop this skill consider:

1. Asking non-directive questions utilizing who, what, where, when, or why such as: "I'm not quite sure I understand what you are saying" or "When you said... what did you mean?"
2. Asking for repetition especially if you are unclear about the child's cause and effect explanation.
3. Summarizing what you heard the child say and seeking feedback such as: "Is this what you meant....?"

Talk about biases. Children need to understand how their emotions, beliefs, and experiences influence their choices. The way we respond to and interpret our emotions, beliefs, and experiences has a major impact on our choices and behavior. When we discuss this issue with parents, we often begin by pointing out that I can call you *careful* or I can call you *slow* in response to the very same behavior. The former implies my positive view, the later my negative or critical view. As the recipient of my comment you will respond very differently depending upon what I say and I will proceed to act very differently. Sometimes, even a careful worker has to speed up!

Belief is a valuable ally in the absence of fact. Unfortunately, human beings often adhere to their beliefs even when fact proves otherwise. As we have written, this is not unexpected given the role Simultaneous Intelligence plays in defending our choices. Children need to learn to guide the application of their Simultaneous Intelligence when facts are available and to judiciously consider alternative actions. Emotional development is a complex process that begins in infancy and continues into adulthood. In this process, parents play a pivotal role in what they do and say. In your everyday interactions with children, you must consistently and frequently help children learn what feelings and emotions are; understand how and why they happen; accurately recognize their feelings and those of others; and develop effective ways of managing them. We must also help children understand how their emotions and experiences contribute to the creation of certain biases and beliefs that may or may not be accurate.

Don't confine critical thinking to purely factual or academic matters. Encourage kids to reason about ethical, moral, and public policy issues. Stephen Kramer and his group at Bright Horizons point out a set of exercises to improve critical thinking ability that makes sense to us. Here are some of their tips and ideas:

Provide opportunities for play. Testing how things work informally is crucial to developing critical thinking. It is during play that children explore cause and effect. What happens if I drop a spoon over and over again off the side of a high chair tray or roll two marbles down a chute at the same time? How can I get the block to balance on the top of this tower? By providing indoor and outdoor space for playing, along with time for pretend play, you provide open-ended opportunities for your child to try something and see the reaction; and then to try something else and see if he can create a different reaction. These hands-on experiences provide an integral foundation for later abstract critical thinking.

Pause and wait. Offering a child ample time to think, attempt a task, or generate a response is critical, but not necessarily easy to do. Try counting (silently) to 60 while your child is thinking, before intervening or speaking. This gives your child a chance to reflect on her response and perhaps refine, rather than respond with her very first gut reaction.

Don't intervene immediately. Instead, observe what your child is doing before stepping in. As challenging as it may be, avoid completing or doing the task for your child. For very young children, patiently readjusting and maneuvering to grasp a toy on their own encourages continued problem solving and develops effective executive functioning.

For older children, ask critical thinking questions such as: "What's happening?" "Why is it important?" or "How do you know?" Provide enough information so children don't get frustrated, but not so much that you solve the problem for them. In short, the goal of critical thinking questions is more than just understanding something; they involve evaluation, critiquing, and developing a depth of knowledge. This type of problem-solving requires creativity, seeking plausible reasons, and a refusal to accept anything at face value.

Ask open-ended questions. Rather than automatically giving answers to the questions your child raises, help him or her think critically by asking questions in return: "What ideas do you have? What do you think is happening here?" Respect his responses whether you view them as correct or not. You could say, "That is interesting. Tell me why you think that." Use phrases like "I am interested to hear your thinking about this." "How would you solve this problem?" "Where do you think we might find more information to solve this problem?"

Help children develop hypotheses. Taking a moment to form hypotheses during play is a critical thinking exercise that helps develop skills. Try asking your child, "If we do this, what do you think will happen?" or "Let's predict what we think will happen next."

Encourage thinking in new and different ways. By allowing children to think differently, you're helping them hone their creative problem-solving skills. Ask questions like, "What other ideas could we try?" Encourage children to generate options by saying, "Let's think of all the possible solutions."

There are situations where as a parent you need to step in. At these times, it is helpful to model your critical thinking. As you work through a decision-making process, verbalize your thoughts. Children learn from observing how you think. Taking time to allow children to navigate problems is integral to developing their Simultaneous Intelligence.

An Old Lion and a Shrewd Fox

There is a fable about an old lion and a shrewd fox. The fable tells the story about a lion, too old to hunt on his own, who instead begins living in a cave and talks to the other animals as they walk by about what wonderful, tasty food he has in the cave. The animals seeking sustenance enter the cave and become dinner for the old lion. One day, a shrewd fox comes by. The lion tries to lure the fox into the cave, but before the lion can finish speaking, the fox notices that there are only footprints of other animals leading into the cave and none leading out. The shrewd fox employed his Simultaneous Intelligence to evaluate all available facts before him. The shrewd fox smiles at the old lion and tells him that some other animal will have to be the lion's dinner for tonight but not him.

Simultaneous Intelligence may be a complex concept to understand; yet it is among the most important instincts that humans possess and can be effectively nurtured in all children. As we have learned, the development of our instincts including Simultaneous Intelligence are dependent upon diverse experiences over a long period of time.

Chapter 7
Genuine Altruism

In Chapter 2, we defined Genuine Altruism as an unselfish concern for and support of others. Throughout this book, we have emphasized that all seven instincts comprising *Tenacity* are interwoven. Genuine Altruism is closely aligned with Compassionate Empathy, given the latter's focus on taking action to alleviate the distress of others. Genuine Altruism places the spotlight not only on lessening distress in others but also on actions taken to enrich their lives even when distress is not present. The word "genuine" captures our belief that altruistic behavior on the part of children is not predicated on their receiving a concrete benefit or reward.

A body of research, especially studies conducted by Psychologists, Drs. Michael Tomasello and Felix Warneken, provide strong support for the genetic basis of altruism and its instinctual expression in children at a very early age. In a 2015 article, published online by the Radcliffe Institute for Advanced Study at Harvard University, author Susan Seligson detailed Dr. Warneken's interest in studying human cooperation as a doctoral candidate at the Max Planck Institute for Evolutionary Anthropology in Leipzig. Dr. Warneken reported that the accepted view at that time was that "the true origin of altruistic inclinations is social norms—that Mother Nature has induced us to be selfish and teachers and parents are always hammering into our heads that we should be empathetic and share. Because of this focus on social norms as the driver of altruism, people often assume that young children, and especially chimpanzees, would never engage in these kinds of helping behaviors."

Dr. Warneken questioned this assumption and asked if altruistic behaviors might be innate or instinctual in very young children. He wondered if toddlers could understand when someone required help. Dr. Warneken wrote that several of the more senior scientists thought it unlikely that toddlers could or would be helpful to others. Perhaps with some amusement, he added, "What did I know? I was just a Ph.D. student."

© Springer Nature Switzerland AG 2021
S. Goldstein and R. B. Brooks, *Tenacity in Children*,
https://doi.org/10.1007/978-3-030-65089-6_7

A Dropped Ball: An Advance in Evolutionary Psychology

Then one day while involved in an unrelated study, Dr. Warneken accidentally dropped a ball. A toddler in the room picked up the ball and handed it to him. As Ms. Seligson noted, once the toddler engaged in that unexpected behavior, it "sent evolutionary psychology hurtling in a fresh new direction." The unexpected reaction of the toddler served as a catalyst for Dr. Warneken to undertake a series of experiments to study the roots of altruism.

In a paper presented at Boston University in 2010, Dr. Warneken detailed different situations he devised for 18-month-olds that involved an adult experiencing difficulty achieving a concrete goal. In an initial study, an experimenter used clothespins to hang towels on a line. In doing so, he "accidentally" dropped a clothespin on the floor and his attempts to reach it were unsuccessful. Another condition involved the experimenter trying to put a stack of magazines into a cabinet, but he was unable to open the door since he had an armful of magazines.

At the Boston University presentation, Dr. Warneken summarized the findings from these and other studies, all of which supported his original hypothesis that altruistic behavior was an innate quality or what we have labeled in this book as an instinct. He stated, "Children displayed spontaneous, unrewarded helping behaviors when another person was unable to achieve his/her goal and did so across a variety of different contexts. Importantly, children performed these behaviors significantly less often in control situations where no help was necessary. This shows that children can differentiate between accidental and purposeful acts and help accordingly."

The results of these experiments prompted Dr. Warneken to ask another question. What would be the impact of introducing a reward to children when they demonstrated helping behaviors? He noted, "Using a crucial distinction from motivational psychology, we may ask whether such acts of altruism are intrinsically or extrinsically motivated." A study published in 2006 with Dr. Michael Tomasello, the co-director of the Max Planck Institute while Dr. Warneken was a student, found that children who were provided with a material reward for helping during an initial phase of the experiment "were subsequently less likely to engage in further helping than children who had not received such a reward."

You may recall that in Chapter 4 we reported a similar dynamic for the instinct of Intrinsic Motivation, namely, that the introduction of a reward for an activity that children naturally enjoyed resulted in diminished enjoyment and a decreased desire to engage in what had been a favored activity. Research findings support the belief that instincts do not derive their nourishment from external rewards but rather from internal or intrinsic forces that fuel their growth and maintenance.

In a series of lectures offered at Stanford University in 2008, and cited by author Adam Gorlick, Dr. Tomasello concluded, "From when they first begin to walk and talk and become truly cultural beings, young children are naturally cooperative and helpful in many—though obviously not all—situations. And they do not get this from adults; it comes naturally."

Dr. Warneken emphasized that "young children are not oblivious to the needs of others. In addition to all of the self-focused and selfish things children do, they can act on behalf of others if the occasion arises. The fact that these behaviors emerge so early in ontogeny suggests that social and moral norms are not the original source of these behaviors. Rather, it appears that cultural factors can build on a biological predisposition we share with our closest evolutionary relatives."

In summarizing a number of their studies in a 2009 article published in the *British Journal of Psychology,* Drs. Warneken and Tomasello, wrote:

> The reported studies demonstrate that human infants and chimpanzees are able and willing to instrumentally help others. With regard to the ontogenetic roots of altruism, these results indicate that children have a natural tendency to develop altruistic behaviors. Socialization practices can build upon this predisposition for altruism, but socialization is not the original source. In other words, we argue against the notion that socialization practices operate independently of an altruistic predisposition or even impose altruism on children who are originally purely selfish. Children appear to have altruistic tendencies as well, and socialization works *in concert with* this predisposition.

Psychotherapist, Mr. Sean Grover also highlighted the benefits of being altruistic in a 2015 article. He observed, "Teaching kids the value of helping others was instrumental in improving their mood and behavior—and reducing bullying. It also roused in them a greater sense of personal worth, a key condition for fostering feelings of happiness and empowerment." Mr. Grover stressed that there was a misconception by some that altruism involved a personal sacrifice, when in fact, "children benefit as much as those they've helped, sometimes even more." To support this statement, Grover cited research that indicated the ways in which altruism reinforced positive relationships with others, a healthier self-image, and a sense of purpose.

Dr. Jonas Miller, a Psychologist and Researcher at the University of California at Davis, studied the physiological impact on a group of four-year-old children when they were engaged in altruistic acts. More specifically, he and his colleagues examined what, if any, changes, occurred in their nervous systems when they were behaving in an altruistic manner. In a 2015 press release detailing his findings for the Association for Psychological Science, Dr. Miller described this fascinating study. The first phase involved playing with children one by one. Then, it was explained to them that they would earn tokens that they could trade for prizes when their visit was finished.

To record their nervous system response, researchers attached (with parental consent) electrodes to each child's torso to gather information about heart rate and vagal tone (this branch of the nervous system is not under conscious control and is largely responsible for the regulation of several bodily functions at rest). As the report noted, "Vagal tone indicates the influence of the vagus nerve, which connects the brain with other key organs and provides a useful measure of the body's ability to regulate physiological stress responses. High vagal tone is related to feeling safe and calm and has been associated with better physical health, behavior, and social skills among young children."

Near the end of the experiment, all of the children were given the opportunity to donate some of their prize tokens to fictitious ill children whom they were told were ill and not able to come to the lab and earn tokens on their own. Each child's vagal tone was analyzed during three phases of the experiment: the introduction segment, the time when each child made a decision about making a donation, and the conclusion when researchers returned to the room, closed the boxes with the tokens without peeking, and placed everything away.

The findings from this study paralleled those reported by Drs. Warneken and Tomasello while adding a physiological measure to the experiment. The children who donated tokens to help the absent, ill children displayed greater vagal flexibility during the experiment, indicating better physiological regulation. The act of donating was, in itself, associated with higher vagal tone at the conclusion of each child's visit to the lab.

Similar to Mr. Grover's observation about the benefits of altruism to the helper, Dr. Miller emphasized, "We usually think of altruism as coming at a cost to the giver, but our findings suggest that when children forgo self-gain to help people who are less fortunate, they may get something back in the form of high vagal tone. This means we might be wired from a young age to derive a sense of safety from providing care for others." The notion of being hardwired from a young age supports our position that Genuine Altruism can be understood as an important instinct present from birth.

Finally, renowned Neuroscientist Dr. Richard Davidson, Founder and Director of the Center for Healthy Minds at the University of Wisconsin at Madison, has also called attention to the impact of altruism on our physiology, including the functioning of the brain. In a 2016 article he wrote, "There are now a plethora of data showing that when individuals engage in generous and altruistic behavior, they actually activate circuits in the brain that are key to fostering well-being. These circuits get activated in a way that is more enduring than the way we respond to other positive incentives, such as winning a game or earning a prize."

It seems apparent that being given a prize for displaying altruistic behavior has little of the impact or staying power that the actual act of altruism provides.

Nurturing Genuine Altruism in Our Children

Similar to the other six instincts, the question that arises is how can parents and other caregivers nurture the biological predisposition that children possess to behave in an altruistic way? As we have emphasized, parents serve as the initial and primary models for their children. The research findings of Drs. Warneken and Tomasello indicate that even in the absence of adults modeling altruistic behavior, 18-month-olds engage in such behaviors. However, it is our conclusion that Genuine Altruism will be reinforced and sustained when children witness the significant adults in their lives not only acting altruistically but in addition, exhibiting enjoyment at doing so.

The following are questions we encourage you to reflect upon that are specifically related to your role of modeling Genuine Altruism and to identify such behaviors in your children:

"What is one example I remember as a child in which I was the recipient of Genuine Altruism and what were my feelings and thoughts at the time?"

"What behaviors have I observed in my children that represent Genuine Altruism and at what age did they show these behaviors?"

"When my children displayed Genuine Altruism, what emotions did they exhibit while engaged in the activity?"

"What do my children observe me saying and doing on a regular basis that models Genuine Altruism?"

"What family activities do I engage in with my children that involve Genuine Altruism?"

These kinds of questions served as a prominent part of our counseling efforts with parents Sy and Jean Lester. They came to see us because of struggles they were having with their two children nine-year-old Hannah and seven-year-old Angie. Jean spoke first. "I know that Hannah and Angie are still young, but there some behaviors that Sy and I are concerned about. Before we know it, they'll be teenagers and most likely when they are, their problems will become even more intense. We want to see if we can head off some of these problems."

We asked, "What problems are you most concerned about?"

"It hurts to say this," Jean replied, "but one of the main issues is that both girls never seem to want to help, whether it's to clean up their rooms or bring their dishes to the dishwasher or anything. Just yesterday I picked them up at a playdate at a family who has girls their age. I was coming straight from the supermarket and there were some grocery bags in the car. Both girls jumped out of the car and neither offered to bring even a small bag into the house. When I asked them to carry one bag each, they said they were tired. Then Hannah asked if she could stay up later if she took a bag in and when Angie heard this, she asked for the same thing. It was very discouraging. Finally, they each took a bag but seemed to resent doing so."

Sy added, "As Jean said, they're young, but you would think that they would know enough to offer to help out. We shouldn't have to remind them and then be met with a demand for a reward such as being allowed to stay up later. I'm concerned that if this continues, they'll become more and more self-centered and expect to get rewards for everything they do. I must admit that I'm feeling resentment towards the girls and I think Jean feels the same."

It's not surprising that parents want their children to be helpful without constant reminders and requests for rewards. However, these seemed to be hot button issues for the Lesters. As we were to discover during our first three sessions with them, their thoughts and behaviors were heavily rooted in their unhappy experiences as children and their efforts to travel a different path than they had experienced with their parents.

Both Sy and Jean described growing up in homes that were emotionally distant. Neither of their sets of parents were perceived as demonstrating affection toward each other or toward them. Sy reflected, "People say opposites attract, but in many ways Jean and I had similar childhoods with both sets of parents expressing little if any love or consideration toward us. I know that by the time I became a teenager and my parents asked me to do something, I often found excuses not to do it. They would tell me I was selfish and bring up something like they drove me to a sporting event, and if they could go out of their way for me, I should be eager to help them. Each time they said something like that, I would get angry and after a while I asked them to do fewer and fewer favors for me."

What became apparent in our discussions with the Lesters is that in their efforts to become better parents to their daughters than they perceived their parents having been toward them, they attempted as Sy realized "to bribe our daughters into being nice, kind people." They did so even as they recalled viewing acts of altruism from an early age in Hannah and Angie that were not rooted in being offered or given rewards. Jean observed, "I remember how both of them wanted to help me even when they were toddlers, whether it was sweeping the kitchen or putting things away."

Sy smiled and interrupted, "And I remember when they were probably four and six coming outside when I was raking leaves and they wanted to help. I ended up buying two small kid-sized rakes and they raked leaves with me and they seemed so pleased with their efforts."

Jean listened closely and added, "Although Sy and I really haven't spoken about it, I think that given our own childhoods we so wanted that behavior to continue and were so concerned that it would not that we began to give them rewards for almost every helping behavior they demonstrated. Before long it seemed as if they became little negotiators, selling their assistance for a reward. Now it seems as if our efforts to maintain their generous actions have backfired. I wanted to be such a good mother, but I feel I haven't done a very good job."

Sy nodded in agreement and said, "I wish we could start over with them and avoid the mistakes we made." Their distress at witnessing the negative outcome of their efforts to nurture altruism in their daughters was evident—as was their negative assessment of their abilities as parents.

Our initial goal in replying to their distress was to convey a sense of empathy and understanding given the intensity of their negative self-evaluations. We replied, "Being a parent can certainly be a humbling experience. Sy, we would guess that every parent at some point had the wish to start over again with new information at their disposal. We believe that kids are born with an inborn need to help and you saw that with Hannah and Angie. With hindsight you're aware that giving them rewards for those behaviors wasn't necessary and actually worked against their wanting to be helpful on their own. But given your own experiences as children, it's understandable why you did what you did. You're not the first nor will you be the last parents to have good intentions that don't work out as you would like."

Both parents appeared to appreciate the empathy we conveyed. Jean asked, "Is it too late to change things, to help them be more thoughtful and kinder?"

We answered, "They're only nine and seven. We certainly think there's time for them to change. But as we always tell parents, you'll first have to examine what you can change in yourselves so that your kids will be more receptive to making changes in their own behaviors."

Jean quickly replied, "I'm willing to look at what I can do differently. We're not happy with the way things are going now with the girls and our relationships with them."

Sy agreed, "Like Jean, I want to learn new ways of parenting. I think both Jean and I feel that we haven't been very effective in that role and it's been painful for me to watch Hannah and Angie's behavior. I love them very much, but I find myself getting more and more upset by the way they behave towards us and towards each other."

We commented, "It's obvious that you love them. As we look at ways to improve the situation, we have some questions we want to ask. If you're not certain why we're asking any particular question, please let us know. Your input is essential as we examine ways of modifying the ways in which you relate to Hannah and Angie." To nurture a collaborative relationship with parents we directly encourage their questions and comments about anything we ask. Not surprisingly, we have found parents are more likely to follow through on what they learn in therapy if they feel they have been active participants in the therapeutic process.

Jean said, "We'll let you know if your questions are not clear. Now I'm curious what kinds of questions you plan to ask."

We discussed how kids closely observe our behavior and the ways in which we serve as models for them. We said the goal of the questions we ask parents is to have them consider how kids view what we say and do. We reviewed with Sy and Jean the questions we introduced earlier in this chapter, including:

"What do my children observe me saying and doing on a regular basis that models altruism?"

"What family activities do I engage in with my children that involve displaying altruism?"

Given what both Sy and Jean reported about their childhoods and the dearth of altruism they experienced, we added a very specific question related to the first two questions: "When Hannah and Angie observe the two of us interacting, what if any displays of altruism do they see?"

All three of the questions generated reflection and discussion, none more so than the third that focused on the ways in which the two of them demonstrated helping behaviors toward each other. The conversation that followed was painful at times for them but also necessary to move forwards. They reported that they recognized that they rarely went out of their way to help each other.

As the dialogue progressed, Sy observed, "These discussions have made me aware that I should be much more tuned into being helpful to Jean and to others as well. I think the girls would be able to give you examples of when I was helpful to them, whether with a school project or at one of their sporting events, but unfortunately, I'm not certain they would be able to give you examples of when I was helpful with Jean or for that matter with other family members or neighbors."

He continued, "And I know I can do a better job of expressing appreciation when Jean has stepped in to help out. Not to blame my own childhood experiences, but I didn't witness words of appreciation when I was growing up. You might think that would make me more aware of the importance of being helpful and appreciative, but not having models showing those kinds of behavior has had an impact on my own behavior as a father and husband."

Jean was attentive to Sy's observations and replied, "I could also do a better job of expressing appreciation. I think the girls would benefit from seeing us doing this. It's not that I don't appreciate what Sy does, it's for whatever reason, I just don't say anything." Echoing what her husband expressed, she noted, "Maybe it's because I don't remember my parents ever showing appreciation or for that matter affection."

Jean paused and with insight added, "But that should not be an excuse. If we want Hannah and Angie to change, then Sy and I have to change. We may not have had great models for being kind and generous, but that doesn't mean we can't learn to model that for our daughters. I know that Sy and I love each other and we love our daughters. Although I may not say it, I've often felt that Sy was one of the best things to happen in my life. We have to rely on that love to change what we've been doing."

We complimented the insights that Sy and Jean were showing and provided several suggestions when they spoke with their daughters. This included that they convey the message that we are a family and that they all had to figure out ways for each of them to support and help each other. At our recommendation, Sy and Jean also asked the girls what they would like to see them do differently as parents that would improve things at home.

Sy and Jean thought Hannah and Angie would immediately default to requesting rewards for helping out, including additional TV time and being allowed to stay up beyond their bedtime. At our next meeting with Sy and Jean, they laughed as they recounted what had occurred when they asked their daughters how they as parents could me more helpful. Jean said, "We were great prognosticators. What we predicted is what they said. Angie told us that one way we could be helpful is to allow them more TV time and to let them stay up later. We were prepared for this response and told them that we knew those were rewards we had previously used, but that in the future we wanted to learn ways of helping out that didn't involve rewards being given."

Jean continued, "We tried to add a little levity by telling them that the best reward would be for all of us to get along better. When I said that, both girls rolled their eyes, but at least they didn't say what a silly notion it was."

Sy asked an important question about the new stance they were assuming as parents. "If we have to ask the kids to help us, isn't that forcing them to be helpful rather than their wanting to be helpful on their own. It still seems external, replacing a reward to get them to do something with forcing them to do something."

We agreed, "That's a very good question. Even though, you're putting some, although we don't think much, pressure on them to be kinder and more helpful without receiving any kind of external reward, the hope is that the natural inclination to be helpful will be reinforced and sustained. Also, we believe that the more they observe the two of you being helpful and appreciative towards them and each other, the more those kinds of behaviors will become a natural part of their behaviors. In terms of the last point, how have things been between the two of you?"

Jean answered in a very telling way by taking Sy's hand. "It's getting better. I think both of us are concentrating on improving how we respond to each other." She then smiled and said, "The other day Sy and I kissed in front of the girls and they giggled when they saw us kissing. We asked why they giggled and Hannah said, 'We never see you kiss. Are you like teenagers again?' My heavens, she's only nine and is talking about being a teenager and kissing. I can only imagine what we have in store with two teenage girls in just a few years."

Our sessions with Sy and Jean continued for approximately a year with a decreased frequency after six or seven months. It was a pleasure to observe their motivation to improve their lives and to enhance their role as parents. In one of our last meetings, they proudly reported how the girls on their own suggested baking cookies with Jean and then selling them to raise money for a child in the neighborhood who was undergoing treatment for cancer. They also described how much more helpful the girls were at home.

Is Praise Okay?

"If rewards serve to lessen altruistic behaviors in children, does that mean we should refrain from praising or acknowledging our children when they've been kind and helpful to us or others?" is a question that is often raised at our parent workshops. "Will they just be acting helpful in order to earn our praise or recognition and not because they value the acts of kindness?"

This question is related to our discussion about Intrinsic Motivation in Chapter 4. As we reported in citing the research conducted by Drs. Lepper, Greene, and Nisbett with 3–5-year-old nursery school children, the enjoyment of drawing was diminished when children were advised in advance that they would receive a reward for this activity. Children who were not told about an award in advance but were given one after they finished drawing, continued to display enthusiasm for the task, similar to children who were not promised nor given an award.

The key dynamic, one that we highlighted in Chapter 4, is the presence of what are labeled "contingent rewards," that is, rewards provided only when certain behaviors are demonstrated. The message associated with contingent rewards is, "You will receive a reward but only if you first do this (whatever *this* might be)." As we previously emphasized, contingent rewards may serve a limited purpose in some situations, but multiple studies over many years have shown that such rewards are rarely successful at producing lasting changes in behaviors or attitudes.

A more effective perspective for parents to adopt is to recognize and verbally appreciate signs of Genuine Altruism expressed by their children. Simple comments from a parent or caregiver such as, "I appreciate you helping out," "Thanks for bringing the dishes over to the dishwasher," "That was very helpful," or "When you helped your friends, I could see that they were really grateful for what you did" serve as more potent reinforcers of Genuine Altruism than offering material rewards. Sy and Jean experienced this firsthand. Their attempts to reinforce altruism in their daughters through the use of external rewards backfired since their efforts conveyed the message that helping behaviors were not worth doing for their own right but only if a reward is given. It was not surprising that the girls became master negotiators when asked to help out. The instinctual nurturing of Genuine Altruism was eclipsed by the belief, "What's in this for me?"

In addition to appreciative comments parents and other caregivers can convey toward children, there are many daily opportunities for parents to demonstrate altruistic behaviors that involve few if any words. Earlier in this chapter, we requested that you reflect upon the following question:

"What do my children observe me saying and doing on a regular basis that models Genuine Altruism?"

How would you reply to that question? Remember that even seemingly small gestures can serve as powerful teaching moments for our children that will last a lifetime. When we asked parents about altruistic actions they recall observing in their own parents, here are a few sample responses:

"I remember my dad walking to the corner of a street to help an elderly woman. I asked if he knew her. He said he didn't, but she looked like she needed some help and that's why I went over to her."

"It wasn't just one thing but a number of things that occurred regularly. My mom often volunteered for different committees at our church. As a teenager I often joined her. I especially remember at one Thanksgiving holiday delivering meals to elderly people before we went home for our own Thanksgiving meal. Mom always seemed so happy when she gave the person a meal. It also made me happy."

"Maybe a lot of people do what my parents did. I don't know. They would make certain that they thanked people, whether a UPS driver delivering a package, or someone in a store helping them find something, or the cashier in the supermarket who rang up their bill. I know we should all do those things, but sometimes we forget or take people for granted. My dad once told me that for some people the only compliment they might receive that day or even during that week was the one we just gave. That comment really stuck with me."

"My mom wrote a note to the head of the Department of Public Works in our town to say how much she appreciated what a nice job the plow truck driver did in plowing our street during a big snowstorm. Our street is on a hill and we could easily get stuck if the road wasn't cleared down to the pavement and salted. I was very impressed when she did that. Interestingly, to this day I send brief notes of appreciation—and now it's even easier with email—to the heads of town departments for services they or one of their staff have provided."

"I felt they never took my helping out for granted, whether it was raking leaves or clearing the dishes or babysitting for my younger brother. There was always a sincere thank you."

One Step at a Time

In these difficult times, many children and adults go through their day stressed and pressured by the events taking place around us. As author, Ms. Ana Morris wrote in

2012 "Call someone by name and ask if they would do something for you instead of demanding it. Say please and thank you. Hold the door for someone. Let that car enter your lane. No one else will. Wave thanks to someone that does the same for you." If we should question if a small gesture could have a lifelong impact, let's recall a seemingly minor event that served as a catalyst for the research undertaken by Dr. Warneken. He accidentally dropped a ball, which prompted a toddler in the room to go and pick it up and hand it to him. As Ms. Seligson reported in her article about Dr. Warneken's research, the toddler's unexpected behavior "sent evolutionary psychology hurtling in a fresh new direction."

Dr. Warneken was already heading in that direction when the toddler picked up the dropped ball. In one sense, it's similar to our position about the instincts identified in this book, namely, children are already heading in a direction to more fully embrace these instincts, including Genuine Altruism. Their interactions with their parents and other caregivers will provide the direction and energy for these instincts to reach their full expression.

Chapter 8
Virtuous Responsibility

Not long ago as we were having dinner with friends, the conversation turned to stories about our families and childhood. We progressed to speaking about experiences with our deceased parents, some recalled fondly, some not so fondly. One friend recalled a time that she and her sister were confronted by their father for soiling the ceiling of their bedroom. One day, twenty to thirty quarter size spots appeared on their bedroom ceiling looking like someone had flung oatmeal to the ceiling and some of it had stuck. Their father, a usually calm parent, became quite angry, in part because he had just recently painted their room, including the ceiling. He insisted that whomever was responsible tell him what they had done.

Neither of the girls had done anything wrong, so both denied causing the problem. After a back and forth banter of accusation and denial during which their father became increasingly more angry, he picked up one of the girls' doll houses and smashed it to the floor, telling the girls that if they could not accept responsibility for their behavior he would be back and break another of their toys. Our friend recalled that as soon as he left, she and her sister began gathering their favorite toys and hiding them in the closet. They knew they hadn't been responsible for the problem, but as children did not know what else to do.

After about fifteen minutes, their father came back into the room looking sheepish and apologized. In the interim he had gone up into the attic and discovered that the spots were caused by rain leaking through the roof and then migrating through the ceiling!

This prompted another friend to recall a time when she and her three siblings were confronted by their mother for breaking one of their mother's favorite cups. The cup had been broken by one of the four, unbeknownst to the other three. Pieces of the cup had then been thrown away. Unfortunately, one rather large piece of the cup was missed by the culprit and found by their mother on the floor. In this family, children under ten years old were spanked for their indiscretions as punishment. Children over ten years old were restricted from favorite activities. The friend was twelve years old at the time. Her three siblings were under ten years of age. After being lined up and confronted by their mother, each of the other three denied responsibility. Our

© Springer Nature Switzerland AG 2021
S. Goldstein and R. B. Brooks, *Tenacity in Children*,
https://doi.org/10.1007/978-3-030-65089-6_8

friend commented that she had not broken the cup so she knew one of her siblings was guilty. However in an altruistic effort to save them from a bout of corporal punishment, which she had never liked nor thought very helpful, she stepped forward and accepted responsibility for breaking the cup. She was restricted from watching television and seeing friends for a week. To this day, she noted none of her three siblings has ever admitted responsibility though all thanked her.

As if these two stories of parents at times desperately, perhaps inappropriately, attempting to teach responsibility to their children was not enough, a third friend added that he was the second of four brothers close in age. Their father was a strict disciplinarian. Any indiscretion was typically responded to "with the belt." As they entered their teenage years, the four brothers made a pact. They agreed that if any of them misbehaved or got into trouble, the guilty party would "come clean" to their father so that the other three would not have to suffer the corporal punishment as it was their father's habit of punishing all four if no one accepted responsibility. Our friend commented, "Our plan usually worked quite well although every once in a while none of us actually did anything wrong or knew what Dad was upset about so we would draw straws. Short straw admitted guilt sometimes even before Dad told us what we had done wrong!"

Listening to these stories, one might think that deniability was the instinct and responsibility was a behavior acquired through punitive experiences. However, we disagree. In Chapter 2, we proposed that the instinct of Virtuous Responsibility encompassed several different behaviors. Its close relationship with Compassionate Empathy is evident when we speak of the ethical and moral responsibility we have to enrich the lives of family, friends, and members of our society. Virtuous Responsibility extends beyond this important scope of helping others when it involves our making good decisions, engaging in behaviors that demonstrate that we can be trusted and are accountable for our actions, whatever those actions might be.

We noted that the existing scientific research in supporting the instinctual foundation for Virtuous Responsibility is not as robust as it is for the other six instincts. However, it is our belief that while life experiences, including at times specific instruction, are essential for the maturation of this instinct—as they are for the other six instincts—there exists an instinctual need or drive to act responsibly. We certainly witness this when Virtuous Responsibility is expressed through contributory activities.

We view assuming accountability for one's behavior, which is a significant dimension of Virtuous Responsibility, as rooted in great part in the ways in which parents and other caregivers discipline children in order to nurture the qualities of self-discipline, responsibility, and accountability. As we will detail in this chapter we have witnessed on many occasions the weakening of Virtuous Responsibility in our clinical practices when well-meaning parents fail to hold their children accountable for the actions they take or engage in misguided efforts that work against developing this instinct. When this occurs, children are likely to remain self-centered and rarely display caring, compassionate, or altruistic behaviors. Failure to develop Virtuous Responsibility impacts negatively on the other six instincts as well.

What follows is a summary of our intervention with the parents of one such family. We describe our work in greater detail than with most of the other vignettes in this book since it captures numerous facets of nurturing the instincts of *Tenacity* in children as well as obstacles that sometimes must be overcome. For the sake of clarity, while our actual dialogue with these parents transpired over a number of sessions, we present this story as one extended discussion. We do so to help you more easily identify and understand the ongoing interventions we used to help these parents to become increasingly effective in nurturing Virtuous Responsibility and the other six instincts in their two sons. We also highlight ways to communicate with children that helps lessen well-entrenched behaviors that work against the emergence of *Tenacity*. As you will also see, some of the dynamics we describe parallel those of the Lester Family whom we highlighted in the previous chapter.

A Portrait of a Family in Distress

Tim and Maryanne Fields contacted us at the recommendation of Chip's school counselor. Chip, a third grader, was struggling in school and had recently been evaluated, resulting in the identification of dyslexia and qualification for Special Education services. However, what prompted the referral from the counselor were her concerns about Chip's immaturity and his parents difficulty setting limits and consequences. The counselor noted, "Chip has difficulty relating to the other kids. He often acts silly and frequently says school is dumb. I know part of that has to do with his learning problems, but he often whines and blames the work."

She continued, "You'll find that the Fields are caring, well-meaning parents, but they seem lost in terms of setting limits. I think whatever Chip wants, he gets. They have a younger son, Will, in first grade. He's doing okay in school, relates more appropriately to his classmates than Chip, but I sense that the Fields are starting to have some of the same problems setting limits with him as they have with Chip."

During our first meeting with Maryanne and Tim they immediately expressed frustration and confusion about how to be what they called "effective" parents. We wondered what they meant by "effective." Maryanne replied, "We want to find ways for our boys to listen to us when we ask them to do something like putting away their toys that they just played with or not throwing their dirty clothes on the floor or putting away their clean clothes in their drawers. They just don't seem to be responsible. Chip is worse than Will, but Will seems to be learning bad habits from his brother."

Tim added, "They're only eight and six, but they seem to be the bosses in the house, deciding what they will or will not do. We can ask them to do something a dozen times. After a while it's just seems easier for us to do whatever we asked them to do."

We inquired, "Do Chip and Will know the specific things you're asking them to do?"

Tim responded, "I think we're very specific, at least most of the time. We'll say to them that they have to pick up their toys in the family room and put them in the toy chest or that they have to put their dirty clothes in the laundry bag."

"Could you give us an example. What exactly happens when you ask them to pick up their toys?"

Maryanne replied, "It's exhausting. We'll say please pick up your toys. Chip will answer that he's busy doing schoolwork when obviously he isn't or he'll start to argue that there's no reason why they have to pick up the toys since they're going to play with them tomorrow. Sometimes, he'll just walk out of the room as if he didn't hear what we had to say. As I said, it's so exhausting that often Tim or I will pick the toys or clothes up. It's just easier for us to do."

Tim chimed in, "Part of the problem, or at least a problem for me, is that Chip has learning problems and sometimes I'm not certain how much pressure to put on him. When Maryanne used the word exhausting, I must admit that I get concerned that Chip comes home from school everyday feeling exhausted. It then takes him so long to finish his homework that I don't want to add one more thing on his plate by asking him to clean up. And then if we don't ask Chip to help out, Will complains that he shouldn't have to help out either. Before we know it, it's up to Maryanne and me to clean up."

We empathized, "Sometimes it can be difficult to know what expectations to have for our kids in terms of helping out, even more so with a child struggling in school. Just to get a clearer view, what responsibilities do Chip and Will have at home?"

Maryanne and Tim looked at each other and shrugged their shoulders. Maryanne said, "At this point, basically none. I mean they're expected to brush their teeth and wash up, but little else. As I'm telling you this, I hope it doesn't sound like we've been terrible parents. We love our boys, but we've struggled helping them to be more responsible. Also, as Tim will probably mention, he especially has trouble saying no to them."

We asked, "What do you mean?"

Tim said, "If we pass a toy store in the mall and they want a toy, I'll tell them that we didn't come to the mall to buy toys. Sometimes I warn them in advance that we're not going to buy a toy. It doesn't matter. Once we're at the mall Chip will keep asking and asking and pleading and pleading and finally I say okay. He is insatiable. No matter how much he has, he wants more. Its not surprising that Will copies his behavior as well. It's hard for me to turn them down."

"What makes it hard? What do you think would happen if you turned them down and did not buy a toy?"

Tim glanced at Maryanne. "Maryanne and I have talked a lot about this. I'm busy growing a business and have to work late many evenings. By the time I get home the kids are already asleep. I feel guilty when I work late and it's up to Maryanne to get them to bed. I also feel guilty that I'm not as available to the kids as I would like to be. I had a really strained relationship with my father and I don't want the same thing to happen between me and my boys. It may sound foolish, but I guess I'm concerned that if I say no to them, they'll resent me. When I tell them I won't buy them a toy or anything else, they immediately say, 'You don't love me. If you loved me, you would buy what I want.' If I continue to say no, they continue to ask over and over again for whatever it is that they want. We used the word exhausting and that's what it is. Eventually I give in. I know it's not the best thing to do, but it calms things down and it stops them, especially Chip, from accusing me of not loving him."

Maryanne said, "This happened just a couple of days ago. Tim took the boys out to get ice cream and when they returned they each had a toy. I must admit that I've done the same thing on occasion, but with Tim it's a more regular occurrence. Sometimes it just seems less of a hassle to give into them."

Ghosts from the Past Impact the Present

Maryanne and Tim's numerous examples of theirs and their sons' behaviors confirmed Tim's earlier observation that Chip and Will "seemed to be the bosses in the house." As the conversation continued, one of the roots of Maryanne's struggles to encourage responsibility in her sons and, in addition, to establish limits on certain behaviors, emerged. She recounted with much emotion the harsh disciplinary techniques imposed by her parents when she was a child, as well as what she considered to be their unrealistic expectations for her "to succeed in all areas of her life." She voiced, "My parents were more concerned about my accomplishments than how I actually felt or what I was interested in. I always felt that the more I accomplished in the areas they considered important like my getting A's in school and excelling in sports, the more it would make them look like good parents to others. I remember the first time as an adult I read about 'conditional love,' and all I could think of was that my parents' epitomized that kind of love with me."

Maryanne then related these experiences as a child with her parents to her behavior as a mother. "I didn't want Chip and Will to see me the same way I saw my parents. As Tim told you, he had a difficult relationship with his father and feels guilty about staying at work until late in the evening and not being home as much as he would like for our sons. I realize that much of what I do as a mother is to avoid Chip and Will seeing me as harsh and as uncaring as I saw my parents. I find it sad and frustrating that in our attempts to be better parents than our parents, we've gone too far over and not held them accountable for what they do or don't do."

It was evident that during the past year Maryanne and Tim had become increasingly upset by theirs and their sons' actions, prompting them to begin to examine in closer detail their parenting styles. Given their uncertainty and distress about what changes they needed to undertake as parents, they actually welcomed the suggestion by the school counselor to contact us. We've observed the difficulties that Maryanne and Tim were experiencing with many well-meaning parents who, in a quest to gain their children's love, became susceptible to lowering reasonable expectations and limits and not holding their children accountable for meeting responsibilities. Not surprisingly, such a parenting approach stunts the growth of Virtuous Responsibility.

It's important to remember that the development of Virtuous Responsibility is also compromised when parental expectations are excessive or too demanding and the consequences for certain behaviors are too harsh. When children feel forced into taking on particular responsibilities and to fulfill unrealistic expectations set by parents—as Maryanne experienced with her parents—there is likely to be a negative impact on the maturation of all seven instincts of *Tenacity*, most noticeably Intrinsic Motivation, Compassionate Empathy, and Virtuous Responsibility. The enjoyment that children typically experience with the full expression of these instincts is lost in a household dominated by the negative emotions that pervaded the Fields' home.

Considering a New Parenting Approach

After Maryanne lamented about the unintended consequences of her and Tim's parenting approach, we interpreted her observation as a desire to consider new parenting strategies that they might adopt. We commented, "It can be very frustrating when parents have good intentions and yet things seem to go off track. It's obvious that both of you want to have a loving relationship with Chip and Will and you also want them to become more responsible and accountable. One of our goals in working with you is to consider the best ways to achieve these goals."

Maryanne said, "I appreciate what you just said. We've tried very hard to be good parents and we do want to figure out the best way to do that since what we've been doing hasn't been very effective."

Our work with Maryanne and Tim encompassed several notable themes. In the remainder of this chapter, we will highlight these themes, all of which involved them becoming more effective parents in reinforcing Virtuous Responsibility, self-discipline, and resilience. In establishing a foundation for our work with the Fields and assisting them to feel more comfortable in setting limits and following through with consequences, we conveyed an essential message, namely, that children actually feel safer when parents set realistic guidelines and consequences for their behaviors and hold them accountable.

In a lighter mood we cautioned that when parents adopt this approach, they should not expect that their children will suddenly say to them, "We know that when you set limits and ask us to do certain things such as clean our room, it's because you love us and you're teaching us to be more responsible. Thus, we want to thank you and let you know we will go along with all of your requests." Of course, we also caution parents that if children actually uttered these words, they should worry about what their children are up to!

Humor when applied at the right time and with respect can be very effective in lessening tense moments. Our intent in introducing a little levity is for parents to be more receptive to hearing a serious message. We emphasize that being a "good" parent requires that we learn to tolerate our children becoming temporarily upset or angry with us when we set limits or ask them to fulfill certain responsibilities, especially if we know that these limits and responsibilities are fair, reasonable, and within their capacity to accomplish. Parents burdened by uncertainty and guilt, as

Maryanne and Tim were, sometimes become almost paralyzed when they attempt to establish and follow through on guidelines and consequences.

To prepare parents to apply new scripts for interacting with their children, we have found it helpful not only to offer some concrete suggestions on what they might say but in addition to anticipate their children's possible responses. This "preparation" with parents includes the communication of several important messages that may appear obvious but are necessary to overcome possible barriers that may occur as parents seek to reach new goals. One message we often convey is not to attempt to modify one's entire parenting style and expectations all at once. Instead, it's more judicious to select even one challenging child behavior upon which to focus. A second point, which many parents reported is very helpful, is not to expect that a change in their behavior will immediately result in a change in their children's behavior. We even "warned" parents that sometimes a child's behavior might worsen in response to the changes parents are making—almost as if the child is testing the parent's resolve to stay the new course.

Rehearsing Setting Limits

With these points in mind, we discussed steps Maryanne and Tim might initiate when Chip and Will continue to demand a toy after they were told in advance that they would not receive such a gift. In our sessions with them we "rehearsed" a new script that they could adopt in their interactions with their sons. Such rehearsals often prove very effective. Parents struggling to modify their approach with their children are more optimistic about the outcome of their efforts when they possess a specific understanding of what to say. Maryanne and Tim enjoyed this role-playing. They learned to communicate to their sons that regardless of how many times they asked or screamed for a present that the answer would remain "no." They also rehearsed that if the boys persisted, they would say in a calm voice, "It's time to go home now." As any parent can attest, as simple as this action might seem, it's easier said than done. However, with our encouragement, they persisted on their agreed upon path, with what Tim described "a few lapses" from time to time.

Not surprisingly, Chip and Will brought up the "you don't love me" card. Maryanne and Tim were well prepared and answered, "We're sorry you feel that way. We do love you, but that doesn't mean we'll buy you everything you want." Tim informed us with some delight that to "spice things up a little," they began to add other comments to their scripted lines such as, "Hopefully at some point some of your love will return." Maryanne reported, "We actually anticipated Chip's reply, 'No, I won't love you ever again.' We calmly said, 'That's up to you, but maybe at some point things will change.'"

"Do You Think We're Nagging You?"

Tim and Maryanne also predicted that Chip would accuse them of nagging him when they reminded him to do something. They wondered how they might respond to this accusation. We replied that when nurturing responsibility in children, it's important to provide them with an opportunity to suggest solutions. This reinforces a sense of ownership for their behaviors. As we discussed in Chapter 4 when describing the instinct of Instrinsic Motivation, children are more likely to engage in and follow through with activities in which they felt they have some input. Adhering to this guideline, we told Maryanne and Tim that one of our favorite strategies, which includes a more humorous side and which we also highlighted in Chapter 4, is to beat our kids' to the punch by asking them, "Do you think we're nagging you?"

Almost all parents upon hearing this recommendation look puzzled. As many of them have asserted, "They constantly accuse me of nagging. Why would I ask them that question? I already know what they'll say. Why open up Pandora's box even more?" Not surprisingly, Maryanne and Tim raised that point.

We inquired, "When they accuse you of nagging them, how do you typically respond."

Maryanne replied, "We often say to Chip and Will, 'We wouldn't have to nag you if. you just did what you were supposed to do.'" She smiled, anticipating what our follow-up question would be. "I bet you're going to ask if that response has helped the situation."

We returned the smile and said, "How did you guess? So if you don't mind we might as well ask the question. Is it helpful when you tell them that if they acted the way you wanted them to act, you wouldn't have to nag them?"

Maryanne responded, "No, it certainly hasn't changed their behavior. They still don't do what we ask. But Tim and I aren't certain what to do."

We observed, "Well let us tell you why we suggest asking kids if we think we're nagging them."

Tim expressed, "Please let us know."

"When you ask your kids if they feel you're nagging them and they reply with the predictable 'yes,' instead of saying you wouldn't nag if they met their responsibilities, you might say, 'I'm glad I asked you. I really don't want to come across as nagging. So I'd really like to figure out with you how you and I can meet our responsibilities without any nagging taking place.'"

Both Maryanne and Tim looked skeptical at this suggestion. Tim wondered, "That can really work?"

We said, "Maybe not the first couple of times, but parents have told us that it eventually opens up a dialogue with their kids about responsibilities and how to meet them. And we might add one other related suggestion that parents have told us has proven helpful."

Tim replied, "We're listening."

"That's to say to kids after you've agreed upon certain expectations, 'We think you'll remember to do what's expected of you, just as we'll try to remember what is expected of us, but just in case we should forget, this is how we would like you to remind us.' You would then tell them of a couple of ways you would like to be reminded. And then you can say to them, 'Just in case you should forget to do something, how would you like us to remind you?' Kids are more likely to tell you how they would like to be reminded if you first tell them how you would like to be reminded. And, of course, if they've told you how you should remind them if they neglect to do something, they are less likely to dismiss what you say as nagging since it was their idea of how to be reminded."

Maryanne expressed, "That's a really interesting idea. My first thought is that Chip and Will as young as they are will see right through what we're doing and feel we're using psychology on them or manipulating them and say 'that's a silly idea.' But my next thought is that it might actually work, especially if we also stick to the limits we set."

We smiled, "In one sense what we're suggesting involves using psychological principles, but not to manipulate Chip and Will but actually to help them to become more responsible and self-disciplined. They've become so accustomed to behaving in a certain way and unfortunately, that way has not been helpful to their development. The purpose of the strategies we just reviewed is to change your usual script so perhaps they will change theirs. As we've emphasized, we're not saying these strategies are going to work immediately, but based on our experience with other parents, eventually they have helped change the behavior of many kids."

Virtuous Responsibility, Cooperation, and Contributory Activities

We continued, "There is a related issue we want to discuss with you. We believe that one of the factors that helps kids to become more cooperative and resilient is when we give them opportunities to help others."

Tim interrupted, "I wish they would be more helpful. They seem not to hear us when we ask them to be more helpful, even as we've mentioned, something as simple as picking up their toys or putting their clothes away. That's why Maryanne and I often end up doing it for them."

We said, "We know it can seem so much easier to do things for our kids. When we do there are fewer hassles and the tasks get done. But, let's put ourselves in your sons' shoes. When you do for them what they should be responsible for, what do you think they're experiencing?"

Maryanne replied, "That sounds like such a simple question, but I never quite thought of it in that way. They may think why should we do anything? If we wait long enough our parents will do it for us."

"That seems like a good guess. So we want to pose another question. If you do for them what they're supposed to do, what have they learned from you?"

Maryanne said, "One strong possibility is that they don't have to be responsible for helping out or they don't have to be accountable for what goes on in our house since we're there to bail them out."

"Those are very perceptive observations. Based on everything you've told us, that kind of behavior is not what you want to see in your kids. And we want to add one more dimension to this discussion."

Tim said, "We're eager to hear what you have to say."

"We feel that part of responsibility is not just being accountable for what one does but also being responsible for helping others." We described our perspective about Compassionate Empathy and the belief that children are born with an inner drive to be helpful. This prompted a discussion of how best to cultivate this drive. Maryanne and Tim had become so accustomed to their sons not being helpful that it was difficult for them to remember times when this drive manifested itself.

We advised that a prime message should be, "We need your help" rather than "remember to do your chores." As we have often conveyed to parents, most children, and we might add adults, are not thrilled by doing "chores," but when these chores are posed as ways of being helpful, the level of cooperation is raised significantly. We suggested to Maryanne and Tim that they clearly define what help they need from their sons for things to run more smoothly at home. We said that similar to our suggestion of asking Chip and Will how they would like to be reminded if they forgot to do something (after Maryanne and Tim told their sons how they would like to be reminded), the same approach could be used in terms of agreed upon ways of being helpful. That is, how each member of the family might remind another member should a task to be helpful not be completed.

Natural and Logical Consequences

At this juncture of our parent counseling, we began to share specific discipline guidelines with Maryanne and Tim that we detailed in our books *Raising Resilient Children* and *Raising a Self-Disciplined Child*. As we wrote in Chapter 1 of this book, self-discipline is closely associated with tenacity and resilience. Although Maryanne and Tim had heard the terms "natural" and "logical" consequences, they were interested in gaining a clearer picture of these concepts and how they might be applied to their interactions with Chip and Will.

We expressed that an important parenting task is to help children learn that there are consequences to their behavior and that these consequences are neither harsh nor arbitrary and that they are based as much as possible on discussions their parents have had with them. We observed that natural and logical consequences can be very effective, especially when the situation is not one that threatens the child's safety or the safety of others.

We then explained the differences between natural and logical and how both can serve to help children develop a sense of responsibility and accountability. Natural consequences are those that result from a child's actions; parents are not required to enforce them because they follow naturally from the child's behavior. As an example, we told them what a parent at one of our workshops reported. She described a situation in which her nine-year-old daughter went out to play on a chilly day. This mother engaged in a heated argument with their daughter about wearing gloves. Finally, she realized this was not a matter of safety, that if her daughter's hands got cold, her daughter would either place them in her jacket or come into the house at some point to get gloves. About 30 minutes after going outside, the girl came in and got her gloves, telling her mother that the temperature had dropped very rapidly since she went outside, an obvious face-saving comment that was wisely accepted by her mother.

Another illustration of a natural consequence that we shared with Maryanne and Tim was a situation in which a father bought his son a new baseball glove and some oil to rub into the glove to soften the leather. He told his son that softening the glove would make it easier to catch a ball. His son neglected to do so, and in the next Little League game he dropped two throws, in part because of how stiff the glove was. Motivated by his own and his teammates' disappointment in the two errors, he immediately applied the oil when he returned home after the game.

While logical consequences sometimes overlap with natural consequences, the former typically involve some action taken on the part of parents in response to a child's behavior. We told Maryanne and Tim of parents of an 11-year-old boy who was late in getting ready for school each morning, and then when he missed the school bus, they always rescued him by driving him to school. His tardiness was not the result of disorganization nor inattention but a consequence of his desire to be driven to school by his parents. If disorganization or inattention had been involved, these parents realized they would have to help him with these issues, that by driving him to school for whatever reason, they were contributing to his lack of responsibility and to his continuing to be late. They told their son that if he were not ready when the bus came, he would have a choice of walking to school (a safe 15-minute walk) or staying home. They felt comfortable offering this latter choice since they knew that he wanted to be in school; obviously, the same choice would not be wise if the child did not want to go to school. They also discussed with him how he might ensure that he was ready on time, knowing he was capable of doing it.

Not surprisingly, even with all of these discussions and preparations, their son was late for school. He pleaded with his parents to drive him to school, assuring them it would not happen again, but they remained appropriately firm and he ended up walking to school. His teacher recorded a note that he was tardy. It was the last time he was late for the bus.

Another example we described to Maryanne and Tim is one familiar to many parents. Parents reminded their nine-year-old son to put his bicycle in the garage at the end of the day. They said that if it were left outside, it could easily be stolen or damaged in a rainstorm. They finally grew tired of these reminders and told their son it would be his responsibility to remember. The boy left the bicycle outside, and sadly, it was stolen. The boy was very upset and asked his parents to buy him a new one. The parents did not retort, "We told you so," but instead said to their son that it would be their son's responsibility to take money out of his savings to purchase a new bicycle. They also provided a number of ways for their son to earn some money for the bike, including doing some extra raking of fall leaves.

Having provided these examples, we then examined with Maryanne and Tim the natural and logical consequences they might use to teach their sons responsibility. They immediately came up with two of their own strategies that were to complement our earlier discussions about "nagging" and listing ways to be reminded. One involved telling the boys that the choice was theirs, if their toys were not picked up, the toys would not be available for them to play with the next day. The second strategy was that if the boys threw their clothes on the floor instead of putting them in the hamper, they would remain on the floor and not be cleaned. Although these were two consequences that Maryanne and Tim quickly thought about, they then voiced skepticism about their effectiveness, wondering if their sons wouldn't care if their toys were not available or they didn't have clean clothes. However, they decided to proceed with these two strategies and learn from the outcome of their efforts.

After one "testing" of the toys and two "testings" of the dirty clothes, Chip and Will complained that their parents weren't being fair, adding their old refrain of "you don't love us." Much to the surprise and delight of Maryanne and Tim, they did not resort to more testings. Tim remarked, "I don't know why we didn't set these limits in the past. The consequences we introduced have certainly been more effective than we expected."

The Danger of Low Expectations for Acting Responsibly

We also addressed the implications of Chip's dyslexia diagnosis. We suggested to Maryanne and Tim that while it's always important to take into consideration the struggles a child is facing such as Chip learning to read, it was equally important not to set expectations below a child's ability. We discussed that to expect Chip not to fulfill particular responsibilities might actually convey the message to him that they did not believe that he was capable of handling these responsibilities successfully. Such a situation could result in a mindset filled with self-doubt and prompt a child to back away from, rather than confront, challenges and responsibilities. We assured them that if they discovered that certain expectations were beyond Chip's abilities, they could modify those expectations rather than rush in and complete them for him. In addition, we felt that the responsibilities they had mapped out were well within Chip's abilities.

Related to Chip's struggles with reading was another prominent dynamic we discussed, namely, his propensity for failing to assume responsibility for improving his reading knowledge and blaming others for his struggles to learn. This lack of accountability could be traced to Chip believing that he was not very smart and his lack of faith that he would ever learn to read effectively. Rather than adopting a more constructive way of coping such as accepting assistance from a reading tutor, he dealt with his self-doubts and sense of helplessness by saying "reading was dumb" or the "teacher wasn't a good teacher."

Maryanne and Tim wondered how best to encourage Chip to take greater responsibility for his learning and to be more accountable for what transpired in school. We offered our perspective that Chip's seeming lack of responsibility was in great part his way of coping with a situation that he felt could not be changed, namely, that he would never learn to read. In addition, he perceived school as an environment that placed the spotlight on his deficits rather than on his strengths. We observed, "It's more daunting to take responsibility for a situation if you believe there's nothing you can do to improve it. A loss of hope often triggers a wish to escape from rather than confront a problem."

Maryanne and Tim questioned if anything could be done to revive hope in their older son. We proposed a number of possible interventions to help Chip experience school and reading in a more positive way, noting, "We believe he will be more willing to accept reading help if he feels more comfortable in school and if he believes that it's possible for him to improve his reading skills. Just telling him that he can learn to read, although it may sound encouraging, is not going to be effective as long as he continues to feel so defeated."

Interventions to Strengthen Hope in the School Setting

We returned to our earlier discussion about "contributory activities" and ways to introduce this strategy in the school setting with the input and assistance of the school counselor. Two specific activities were initiated, one involved Chip helping a school custodian to clean up after lunch for about 10 minutes. Chip liked this custodian. The custodian liked Chip and was complimentary about his work. He would tell Chip that he was pleased that he met his responsibilities without having to be reminded. The latter comment was very reassuring to Chip's parents—one source of evidence that Chip could learn to be more responsible. In addition, this work with the custodian provided an initial source of positive emotions in the school setting.

The second activity was one we have used with many students with learning problems. Chip was asked to read very short stories to two kindergarten students twice a week for 10 minutes. Three other students in his class were asked to do the same with other pairs of kindergarteners so that Chip did not think he was being singled out. He and the three peers in his class were informed by his teacher that the kindergarten teacher would "love having an older student read to students in her class."

Chip was hesitant at first to accept this invitation, most likely a result of his negative feelings about being a poor reader. However, when he was shown the book he would read, he realized that he could read all the text. He quickly came to enjoy this activity, especially given the enthusiastic response of the two kindergarten students when he came to read to them. A direct benefit was that reading began to be associated with positive emotions and he became increasingly willing to accept reading tutoring for himself. The tutor couched her work in part as a way of helping Chip to become a more effective reader so that at some point he could read "higher level" books to his kindergarten twosome.

We saw Maryanne and Tim on a weekly basis for more than a year. As things improved, we shifted to every other week and then once a month. The Fields found it helpful to stay in touch and provide an update every few months for several years. We encourage parents to periodically send us updates and questions via email. We have found that email is an effective way for parents to share their concerns about their children and also the achievements they have observed. In addition, retaining and re-reading the emails over several years helps to place a spotlight on the advances that have taken place. The Fields reported that except for some brief "hiccups," for the most part things were progressing in a smooth fashion since we last saw them. They believed that they had become more effective parents and that Chip and Will had become more responsible, caring children.

A Brief Summary of Our Interventions

We wrote earlier in this chapter that we decided to describe our interventions with Maryanne and Tim in greater detail than other vignettes in this book since the topics captured a number of very specific strategies for strengthening not only the instinct of Virtuous Responsibility but several of the other instincts as well. To summarize, we covered the following five key points in describing the actions required for Virtuous Responsibility and all the instincts of *Tenacity* to be nurtured. Take a few minutes as you read each below and think of two or three ways that you can reinforce these in your family.

1. Communicating realistic expectations to your children.
2. Creating opportunities for your children to learn to be responsible and account-able for their actions as well as not blame others when their responsibilities are not fulfilled.
3. Providing experiences for your children to learn that being responsible also involves enriching the lives of others (a feature closely aligned with Compassionate Empathy).
4. Modeling for your children that even if experiencing fear in the face of obstacles or setbacks, they continue to pursue goals and responsibilities, and perceive such challenges as opportunities for growth and learning.
5. Employing forms of discipline that promote self-discipline and responsibility in your children by relying on techniques such as natural and logical consequences.

Four People

There is a fable about four people named Everybody, Somebody, Anybody, and Nobody. There was an important job to be done and Everybody was asked to do it.

Everybody was sure Somebody would do it, so he didn't. Anybody could have done it, but then Nobody did it. Somebody got angry about that, because it was Everybody's job. Everybody thought Anybody could do it, but Nobody realized that Everybody wouldn't do it. It ended up that Everybody blamed Somebody when Nobody did what Anybody could have done!

As this fable illustrates, Virtuous Responsibility is a complicated instinct defined by many variables. As one child with whom we worked commented, "I'm happy to tell everyone when I do something good, but when I do something bad why would I want anyone to know, I'll just get grounded." We all are prone, at times, to associate avoiding responsibility with avoiding negative consequences. If you truly understand the positive nature of Virtuous Responsibility, you can lessen the possibility of your children developing negative associations with being responsible and accountable. Instead, you can nurture this instinct in the healthy ways we have described.

Chapter 9
Measured Fairness

In Chapter 2, we asked how often have you heard children protest, "But that's not fair!" or "He got more than I got!" or "You let her stay up later than you let me stay up!"? In many households, the answer from often frustrated parents is "I hear these complaints on a daily basis." One mother at our workshop observed in a humorous way, "If I didn't know better, I would think there is a 'fairness gene.' I think the first words my kids used when they began to talk weren't 'mommy' or 'daddy' but rather 'it's not fair.'" Although she may have been kidding when suggesting the existence of a fairness gene, she may not have been wrong about the inborn quality of a child's sense of fairness.

One of the authors (Bob) remembers that when he and his twin brother Michael were very young children, their mother brought over glasses of water for both of them at mealtime. Bob observed, "We would move the glasses next to each other to determine if one had received more water than the other. We were keenly observant if one of us had received less and would verbalize the inequality to our mother. Our mother would remind us that the water was freely dispensed from the faucet and she could get more water for either of us at any time. Her logic did not dissuade us however, from continuing to compare water levels with an eye on fairness."

Humans aren't the only ones who cry "no fair." At the Neuroscience Institute and the Language Research Center at Georgia State University, researcher Sarah Brosnan has spent the last decade studying how social animals like primates make decisions, in particular their behavioral responses to equal versus unequal compensation. Among the most intriguing of these studies is her work with Dr. Frans deWaal of the Yerkes National Primate Research Center at Emory University involving capuchin monkeys. Two capuchin monkeys, who deem cucumbers a fine reward, but much prefer sweet grapes, are asked to do a simple task. The first monkey performs the task and happily receives her reward, the cucumber. Immediately, she notices that the second monkey receives the preferred grape after doing the same task. "That's not fair" she must be thinking. When she again receives the cucumber, she resorts to unabashed protest by howling and violently jiggling the bars of her cage to rattle the experimenter to hear her complaint. After this sequence is repeated, she again howls and as a final act of

© Springer Nature Switzerland AG 2021   111
S. Goldstein and R. B. Brooks, *Tenacity in Children*,
https://doi.org/10.1007/978-3-030-65089-6_9

discontent she reaches through the small hole of her cage and vehemently rejects the cucumber by throwing it at the experimenter. She then sees that the second monkey is now the object of the experimenter's attention. Again, the other monkey receives a grape. The first monkey is undaunted in her determination to have her protest heard and continues to howl and bang on her cage. She absolutely can't believe this is happening. This seemingly adorable capuchin monkey has been transformed from a complacent, task-following pleaser to a wild, irreverent, and contemptuous participant. She's visibly undone at the unfairness of it all.

For primates, if you are fair to them, they will be fair to you. Dr. Darby Proctor, a primatologist at Emory University, reported on research with chimpanzees demonstrating that apes will dole out an equitable share of their bananas—and when they don't, the others will complain. At a later point, when the others have food to share, they will not share with the previously selfish member. Reciprocity reigns and exists in other species too. Some bats are known to need a blood-feeding every sixty hours at least. If not, they will die. When their group members see that they have not been fed, they will regurgitate blood feedings to help save lives. However, they will not do so for bats who have not helped in the past. These acts of fairness and the subsequent prosocial benefits are ubiquitous in the animal kingdom.

The universality and intensity of complaints about unfairness, beginning at such a young age, support our belief that measured fairness is a formidable instinct. We use the descriptive word "Measured" to reflect our belief that this instinct goes far beyond fair being judged as always equal such as the level of water in one's glass. Rather, as the instinct of Measured Fairness evolves, its expression becomes increasingly reflective and rooted in all situations experienced by a child or adult for that matter. Measured Fairness, which we view as closely allied to such prosocial behaviors as effective communication, empathy, cooperation, problem-solving skills, and forgiveness, is a basic underpinning of leading a connected, generous, and successful life.

Research examining the nature of this instinct highlights two main findings, both of which are similar to those we reported for the other six instincts. The first is that very young children, even before they can use words, are already attuned to situations they experience as displaying fairness or unfairness. The second is that life experiences, not only within one's family but within one's culture as well, determine the course and manifestations of this instinct during one's life.

A Sense of Fairness: Present from an Early Age

In 2016, Dr. Jing Li, a psychologist at the Chinese Academy of Sciences in Beijing, and several colleagues in the USA noted, "Fairness is one of the most important foundations of morality and may have played a key role in the evolution of cooperation in human beings." They observed that the concept of fairness has not only been studied in child development but in the field of behavioral economics as well.

One dimension of fairness that has received particular attention has been labeled "inequity aversion" (I.A.) by researchers Drs. Ernst Fehr and Klaus Schmidt in 1999 in their theory of fairness, competition, and cooperation. Two forms of I.A. have been studied, one "disadvantageous inequity" (D.I.) that occurs when another individual receives more of a resource than we do. The second is "advantageous inequity" (A.I.) in which we receive more than another person. In reviewing the fairness literature, Dr. Li and her colleagues wrote that children begin to comprehend fairness between the ages of four and six. Four-year-old children were likely to distribute stickers in a selfish manner to a fictitious partner; an obvious shift was already taking place by the time children were five years of age when these youngsters began to distribute stickers in a more equitable fashion.

A further shift occurred by the time these children are six and seven. Not only did this group display the desire to share equally, but when they recognized that they possessed more of something than another person they were willing to relinquish some but not all of what they had to ensure that they did not have more than this other individual. Dr. Li and her colleagues concluded that fairness continues to mature during childhood, basically moving from a more self-centered, selfish perspective to one in which consideration was given to the feelings and thoughts of the other person. Given these findings, one can see how closely involved Measured Fairness is with the instincts of Compassionate Empathy and Genuine Altruism.

While reporting about changes in the experience of fairness in children aged four through seven, Dr. Li and her colleagues emphasized that the roots of fairness could be traced back to a much younger age, citing research conducted with infants and preschoolers that revealed that knowledge of fairness and fair behavior emerged earlier than originally thought. In one study, infants as young as 16 months were already aware of whether or not resources were distributed equally. Another study placed the onset age even a little younger, at 15 months.

Dr. Li noted that difference s found in the ages in which children displayed a sense of fairness might be based on the research paradigms used. One possible factor was that some research focused on knowledge of fairness, while other studies examined behaviors associated with fairness. Knowing what to do does not always translate into doing what you know is the right thing. This dynamic was evident in a series of studies undertaken by Drs. Craig Smith at the University of Michigan, Peter Blake at Boston University, and Paul Harris at the Harvard Graduate School of Education reported in 2016.

Dr. Smith, in an article describing this research, wrote that seven- and eight-year-old children were inclined to share their stickers equally, while younger children were more likely to keep most of the stickers for themselves. However, all of the children asserted that "the stickers *should* be shared evenly." These researchers concluded, "From an early age, children are aware of local norms related to fair sharing, but it's not until age seven or eight that they consistently follow such norms." Another study found that by about eight years of age children in the USA were likely to "follow norms of fairness even when it means having less for oneself."

Dr. Smith also discussed the concept of fairness in the context of other experimental conditions, including the response of children when one person was obviously more deserving of a reward than another person. He cited the work of Dr. Nicolas Baumard in France. Dr. Baumard described two characters to preschool children, one who worked diligently to make a batch of cookies and another who expended little energy in doing so. The preschoolers were given an opportunity to disperse three cookies to the two characters in any way they wished to do so.

The most common response was for these preschoolers to give one cookie to the hard worker and one to the one who slacked off, which meant that the third cookie was not given to either character. When encouraged by the experimenter to hand out the third cookie, nearly 70% offered it to the hard worker. Dr. Smith commented that young children appeared to comprehend that some individuals may be more deserving of receiving a reward than others, but they still preferred to distribute rewards equally if given the opportunity. He added that other studies showed that a preference for "deservingness-based" allocation is even more prominent when children reach middle childhood.

Fairness and Punishment

Drs. Smith and Warneken, the latter whose studies about altruism we described in Chapter 7, questioned if differences in the response of children to fairness extended beyond rewards and to punishments as well. Specifically, they wondered given the results from reward conditions if (a) young children were inclined to dispense punishments out equally regardless of the behaviors involved and (b) older children preferred that punishments be meted out to those whose behaviors warrant such consequences. Their research involved 123 four-to-ten-year-old children being shown classroom situations that captured one student doing more of good or bad things than another student. The same scenarios were shown to a group of 90 adults. As an example of one scenario, a student ignored a teacher's request to take off his shoes, and as a result made a mess, while another student listened to the teacher and did not make a mess.

The four-to-five-year old children were the ones most likely to prefer that both rewards and punishments be given equally to the two people, even if one had displayed more of a good or bad behavior than the other. In contrast, older children and adults favored equitable amounts of rewards and punishments in which good behavior resulted in more reward, while bad behavior earned greater punishment. Dr. Smith concluded, "The developmental shift toward a preference for allocating discipline based on *deservingness*—and away from a consistent preference for equal allocation—is very similar where both rewards and punishments are concerned."

Dr. Smith discussed the implications of these findings for adults interacting with children, especially in terms of the disciplinary techniques that are used. As one example, he noted that a teacher who rewards an entire class for the good actions of one student might be perceived as very fair by young children but as less fair by older children. Relatedly, school age children compared with preschoolers were likely to react more negatively to the practice of punishing the entire class for the misdeeds of one or two students.

Beyond the Family: Cultural Differences

These studies support our position that Measured Fairness, similar to the other six instincts we have described, is inborn and open to continual change in outlook and expression as children develop. Other research found that the determinants of outlook and expression extend far beyond the child's immediate family and involve the child's broader culture. Instincts are not static entities set on a fixed path from birth. Rather, many familial and cultural forces determine the forms they will assume throughout childhood and into adulthood. This situation is evident when one examines research about fairness undertaken in different countries.

Professor, Dr. Peter Blake, a faculty member in the Department of Psychological & Brain Sciences at Boston University, together with colleagues located throughout the world, reported in 2015 on differences in children's fairness behavior in seven countries including Canada, India, Mexico, Peru, Senegal, Uganda, and the USA. To study fairness, the researchers built a toy they called "the Skittle-ator." Two children sat facing each other on either side of this apparatus with a two-foot-long wooden plank with two small raised trays near the center that contained the Skittles candy. In front of one child were two handles, one red and one green. If the child pulled the green handle, the trays tipped toward both children so that each received the candies in their bowls. In contrast, if the child pulled the red handle, the Skittles slid into a bowl in the middle so that neither child received any of the goodies.

Different "deals" were included. When four- and five-year-old children were offered a "good deal" in which the child pulling the handling received four Skittles and the other child one Skittle, the child pulled the green handle and displayed happiness in receiving four Skittles. In contrast, when a "bad deal" was put forth with the child controlling the handles being offered one piece of candy and the other four, most of the children pulled the red handle so that neither child received any of the Skittles.

Dr. Blake observed, "Kids are willing to pay the price to prevent the bad deal and it just becomes stronger with age," but he added that about the age of eight, kids began to reject the "good deal" as well. "When we asked the kids why, they would say, 'It's not fair to the other kid.'" These findings, which are parallel to those described above by Drs. Li, Smith, Baumard, and Warneken, prompted the researchers to advance the following position: "If this trait—refusing a deal that's unfair to others—appears only around age eight, only in humans, and goes against economic models of rationality, something bigger than biology must be at work. This seems like a behavior that is shaped by culture."

The findings of the research conducted by Dr. Blake and his colleagues in seven different countries support the influence of environmental and cultural forces in determining the form and expression of instinctual behavior. In planning the research study, Dr. Katherine McAuliffe, a psychologist on the faculty of Boston College and a collaborator with Dr. Blake observed that an initial study of fairness involved children only from the USA, more specifically from the Boston area. She asked, "But is the developmental trajectory in the United States the same across cultures? What is the true sense of human fairness?"

The scientists hypothesized that children from all seven countries would reject the "bad deal" and that is what they found. However, children from Mexico rejected the bad deal at a much later age than their peers from the other countries, about 10 years of age rather than four. One explanation was that the Mexican children were drawn from a close-knit Mayan community that discouraged competition.

The findings from the "good deal" were not fully predicted. The researchers believed that children in Canada, similar to those in the USA, would refuse the good deal at about the age of eight given the common cultural norms that existed between the two countries. In fact, these two groups of children did respond in this way but so too did the children of Uganda. To explain the Ugandan children's responses, the researchers referred to one possible explanation that they recommended be addressed in future studies. The Ugandan children were basically composed of a specific subset of children in their country with most recruited from schools that had Western teachers—teachers who may have had an impact on the children's views of fairness. Children from the other four countries did not show aversion to receiving more than their peers even when they reached the age of eight.

These researchers cautioned that the results of the study did not necessarily imply that the population in some countries were fairer than others. They noted that follow-up studies should be conducted to examine whether these findings hold true when children reach adolescence. Professor Kristina Olson on the faculty of the University of Washington asserted, "This research makes it clear that while some aspects of a concern with fairness appear to be fairly universal, not all aspects are the same in every place." Psychologist and author Maria Konnikova, in summarizing the work of Drs. Blake, McAuliffe, and their colleagues wrote that while A.I. and D.I. had much in common they appeared to differ in one essential way, namely "D.I. is innate: all over the world, and in the animal kingdom, getting less than others is perceived as an insult. A.I., on the other hand, seems to be a product of social life or culture."

These studies, undertaken in a laboratory setting, examined the concept of fairness primarily through the lens of equitable sharing, whether using stickers, Skittles, or different forms of rewards and punishments. The findings derived from experimental studies are important in identifying the early emergence and expressions of fairness. However, we now turn to another important source of data about fairness, what we have observed many times in our clinical practice.

The Presence of "Why Me?"

As psychotherapists, we have worked with many children, adolescents, and adults who believe that life has been unfair to them and has placed them at a disadvantage in numerous situations. We have especially witnessed this dynamic with patients who are confronted with learning or attentional problems or physical disabilities.

We saw such an instance with Madison in Chapter 3. She is the nine-year-old child diagnosed with dyslexia at the age of six. Her parents, Mia and Joe Salter, were concerned by the increasing frustration and disappointment Madison displayed as she struggled to learn to read even with additional tutoring. Madison told her parents, "I don't know if I'll ever learn to read like the other kids. I wish I never had dyslexia. Why do I have to have it?" The not so implicit message was "it's unfair that I have dyslexia."

A child such as Madison inquiring, "Why me?" or parents wondering "Why my child?" is a very natural response on the part of both children and their parents when burdened with challenges not encountered by others. However, if these questions continue to be asked week after week and year after year without any satisfactory resolution, they reinforce what has been labeled a "victim's mentality" that serves as a formidable roadblock for the seven instincts to blossom.

How do we best manage a "why me?" attitude in a child, especially as a parent or other caregiver? It's important that we adopt a "personal control" outlook and help our children to do the same. We introduced the concept of personal control in Chapter 3 in the context of Instinctual Optimism. It is rooted in the belief that "we are the authors of our own lives" and that while there are events over which we have little, if any, control, what we have more control over than we may realize are our attitude and response to these events. If a personal control attitude is lacking in a child, if a victim's mentality is dominant, it will require skillful communication by parents and other caregivers to change this mentality into one that welcomes hope and constructive action to address the challenging situation.

An illustration of a strong sense of unfairness was evident in 11-year-old Joel. He had one sibling, Jay, who was nine. Joel's parents, Lila and Bret Lancaster, were becoming increasingly concerned about his "sadness" and seeming "lack of motivation" both in school and home. Joel had been diagnosed with Attention Deficit/Hyperactivity Disorder (ADHD) at the age of eight, and in addition to his struggles with attention and impulsivity, he had difficulty processing or comprehending what he was reading. Similar to what Madison's parents experienced in dealing with her defeatist attitude, Lila told us that Joel's favorite comments were "Why do I have to have ADHD? It's not fair." and, more recently and of greater concern to the Lancasters, was his pronouncement, "I wish I was never born, then I wouldn't have to go to school."

Lila and Bret shared another major concern involving Joel's interaction with Jay. Bret told us, "Everything comes easy for Jay whether in school or sports or anywhere. Jay is a really sweet kid and never brags about anything he does. He's never said anything mean to Joel or pointed out that he's reading at the same or perhaps a higher level than his brother. It seems obvious to us that Jay would love to do more things with Joel. The problem is that Joel treats Jay in a horrible way. He constantly taunts Jay, calls him a pest, and doesn't allow him to come into his room. A couple of days ago he told Jay that he was a loser. It's painful to watch what's going on. Lila and I are worried that if Joel continues to treat Jay in this way, Jay probably won't want to have any relationship with him in the future."

Lila added, "Bret and I are not psychologists, but we've discussed when Joel calls Jay a loser, that's probably how he feels about himself. It seems obvious that he resents Jay, not because of anything that Jay has said or done but because so many things seem so easy for Jay, especially in school and sports. Everything seems so much more of a struggle and so much more frustrating for Joel than for Jay and we're certain that's one of the reasons that he puts Jay down."

Bret expanded on Lila's comment. "When I think of the two boys, the picture I have of Jay is always swimming in the same direction as the current is flowing, while with Joel, it's like he's always swimming against the current. Not only doesn't he make any progress, but sometimes he loses ground. It just seems like a constant struggle for him and after a while he must feel frustrated and wonder if things will ever improve."

We empathized with how difficult things have been for Joel as well as for them as they attempt to help him. We also complimented them on their efforts to be empathic in order to better understand how Joel perceives himself and others. As is our practice, we inquired about Joel's strengths or his islands of competence. Bret quickly replied that Joel loved to create structures out of Legos and that he was very proficient in doing so, often without referring to the instructions. Bret smiled and said, "I think he finds looking at the instructions a distraction. When he's ready to begin he'll glance at the picture of the final product and that's it. He rarely looks at the instructions. I don't know how he does it. I would need the directions in front of me every step of the way."

Lila observed that not only was Joel very focused when he assembled a Lego structure, but he also displayed noticeable enthusiasm, sometimes even displaying a smile while working. Then she sadly commented, "If we try to compliment Joel about one of his finished Lego models, even one that includes hundreds of pieces such as a spaceship he did, it seems his default response is to dismiss the compliment, saying, 'It was easy, anyone could build it, even a preschooler.' It gets to the point that Bret and I wonder if we should praise him about anything he does."

Bret chimed in. "Jay also likes to put things together with Legos, but he certainly doesn't have the same Lego skills that Joel does. If Jay gets stuck figuring out how to put some pieces together, he'll look at the instructions and if that doesn't help, he'll ask us for help. One time when we asked Joel to give his brother some help, he yelled, 'He's the smart one, let him figure out what to do. No one helps me when I'm having a problem with something.' What's puzzling and frustrating is that when we've offered to help Joel, especially with his schoolwork, he tells us he doesn't need help and then he accuses us of not helping him. You just can't win."

During our sessions with the Lancasters, we worked with Joel in individual therapy, and with his parents in parent counseling. We also held several family meetings that included Jay at a later point in our work with this family. Given the focus of this chapter, we want to highlight the sessions that pertained to Joel's outlook about fairness and the ways in which that outlook served as a formidable obstacle to his successfully confronting different challenges in his life.

After several months of weekly meetings with Joel, he displayed greater trust and openness. During one memorable session, he looked especially sad. When we commented about how he appeared, he just shrugged. We asked, "Is there something in particular you're sad about? If so, maybe we can help." He responded, "No one can help!" and then lamented, "Why did God choose me to be the one with ADHD?" That statement was quickly followed by, "Jay is so lucky, school is so easy for him. He's already forgotten more than I'll ever learn. It's just not fair!"

In any psychotherapist's career, there are certain sessions that stand out, that vividly capture the inner world of patients, their emotions and thoughts, and that open a portal into gaining new insights that result in new perspectives for both the patient and the therapist. This session with Joel was one of those.

We replied, "We're glad you could tell us how you're feeling, including that you don't think anyone can be of help. We know that right now you don't think things can change or anyone can help, but we just want to offer another opinion for you to think about. We believe that there's a good chance that things can change and that we can help that to happen. We agree that things aren't fair in terms of some kids having an easier time in school than other kids. There's really no great explanation for why some kids are great at some things and not at other things."

Joel listened intently and jumped in, zeroing in on our use of the word *great*, "I don't do anything great."

We repeated our earlier sentiment. "We know that's how you feel right now and we think that's one of the reasons you often feel upset. It's tough to think that you can't learn as easily as other kids or be as good in sports." We paused and then suggested, "By the way, we think we know something you're very good at. Building things with Legos." (In a previous session Joel, at our request, had brought in one of his Lego structures to show us.)

Joel quickly replied, "Yeah, but Legos are easy to do."

"It's easy for you, but for a lot of kids and adults it's not so easy, even if they're looking closely at the instructions that come with the box."

Joel nodded and we continued. "When you asked why God chose you to be the one with ADHD, we can say that we don't know why some kids have ADHD and some don't, but we do know something very important. Do you know what that is?"

"What?"

"That we're learning more and more about the best ways for kids with ADHD to learn and the best ways for educators to teach them. We know it's often more difficult for kids with ADHD to learn some subjects in school and some things outside of school, but we also know that even if it takes them longer to learn than other kids, they can still learn so many things. Sometimes things seem very unfair and it's okay to feel that way. But we think it's also important to think about how to start doing even difficult things. If we don't start, we'll never know what we're capable of achieving."

Joel was truly tuned into what we were saying. As may be evident from our dialogue, our goal was to express empathy for his plight, validate his feelings about things being unfair, introduce the thought that while he had no control over having ADHD, what he had control over was his attitude and response to this condition (a basic assumption of "personal control"), acknowledge his islands of competence, and emphasize our wish to help him.

We are acutely aware as clinicians that mindsets and their accompanying behavioral scripts do not change overnight. However, this particular session was a watershed moment in our therapeutic intervention with Joel and his family. We worked closely with his parents and school to implement teaching strategies that were in keeping with his learning style. One of his teachers, in learning about Joel's ability in building Lego structures, began a Lego club at the school that other students joined, many of whom were not as skilled as Joel. Joel often assisted some of his peers during club meetings, and according to the teacher it was evident that they admired Joel's skills.

The club provided Joel with an opportunity to display his island of competence, to become, as the teacher described, "a source of expertise," and to develop closer relationships with a few peers who were also members of the Lego club. As he formed these relationships over an interest in Legos, his feelings of isolation in school slowly diminished. In one of our sessions, he remarked that it was nice to have some kids say hello to him at school. Adding to the positive changes occurring, a display was created in the lobby of the school with completed Lego models, including Joel's, together with photos of the students who had constructed them. Joel proudly brought in several photos to show us, one with him and his Lego model and another with him and two other students, standing next to their models.

We were involved with the Lancaster family and Joel's school for almost two years, by which time things had improved significantly. Joel had slowly adopted an attitude of personal control, accepting that while he had learning and attentional problems that made it more of a struggle for him to learn than many of his peers, it was not impossible for him to succeed at a variety of tasks. With this perspective, he was more receptive to receiving help in different situations, including therapy, school, and with a tutor outside of school.

Lila described Joel as "being more comfortable in his own skin." She noted as one example that he seemed much happier and less tense in his relationship with Jay. The unprovoked jealousy and anger he had felt toward his brother lessened noticeably as he came to accept that his struggles with learning were not related to anything Jay had said or done. This change in attitude was facilitated when Joel came to appreciate his own islands of competence. Bret commented, "As Lila said, Joel seems more comfortable in his own skin. I think one example is that we're able to compliment him now and instead of dismissing our compliments, he says 'thank you.'"

Reflections on the Futility of Asking "Why Me?"

There are many accounts of individuals who while facing very difficult circumstances recognized that falling prey to an attitude of "It's not fair!" or "Why me?" served as a detriment to leading a more purposeful, accomplished, and caring life. We want to highlight the experience of one such person, the late Christopher Reeve. We believe that his reflections about the way in which his life was drastically altered in one tragic moment and how he coped with that tragedy provide insights for parents as they seek to nurture Measured Fairness in their children while also discouraging the emergence of an "It's not fair!" mentality.

Reeve, an accomplished actor, gained stardom portraying Superman in several movies. At the age of 43 in 1995, he suffered a devastating accident during a horseback riding event. He was thrown from the horse and instantly the "Man of Steel" became a quadriplegic, requiring a ventilator to take even a single breath. In a 2003 interview with Ms. Diane Cyr, a year before he died, he revealed that immediately following the accident he questioned whether it would be better if he had died. In subsequent years, while still struggling with sadness, he adopted a mindset of hope and resolve. He focused not on what he could no longer do but rather on what he still could do, including acting in and directing movies, giving speeches, and becoming a very visible and vocal advocate for research into spinal cord injuries.

A major suggestion that Reeve offered during the 2003 interview was that if you are to move beyond a "Why me?" or "It's not fair!" mindset, it was important "not to look for the reason." Reeve perceptively observed, "People say 'there's a reason' because it allows them to believe life is not chaos, that it's not random. I don't agree with that. I think life is random. I wasn't injured for a reason. I was injured in a freak accident." Very importantly, Reeve did not equate a lack of reason as implying that you cannot derive meaning from a calamity. He emphasized that it's okay to be angry or sad at what has occurred, but then asserted, "After you survive a traumatic event, the challenge is to make sense of it, and then to find a new and perhaps different way of living a meaningful life. I believe one of the key indicators of emotional health is the ability to function well in the present and make plans for the future. I'm able to do that. I can choose to stop thinking, 'I could have been sailing on this day five years ago,' and start thinking, 'What am I going to do today?'"

Reeve continued with this thought-provoking view: "I believe paralysis is a choice. I am literally paralyzed, but in many ways I am free. A lot of people are free of physical limitations, but paralyzed by fear and anxiety, depression, a sense of helplessness. They don't believe their lives will improve. And they're as good as paralyzed."

While most people do not face the tragic event experienced by Reeve, many encounter situations in their lives that occasion the feeling of unfairness, a feeling that can sabotage the development of Measured Fairness. A challenge for parents and other caregivers is to help themselves and their children realize that when difficult events occur, our task is to make sense of these events and recognize that we have more control than we may realize in terms of our attitude and response to the ramifications of that event—a viewpoint so eloquently stated by Reeve.

The "Isms" that Undermine Fairness

The studies reported earlier in this chapter support our belief in the instinctual foundation of Measured Fairness. In the description of our interactions with Joel and his parents, we called attention to factors operating within individuals and families that influence the development of these instincts. The studies undertaken by Dr. Blake in seven countries extended our understanding to include cultural variables as significant influencers of the ways in which instincts are expressed.

Three powerful and what we consider today to be destructive instincts exist alongside the seven instincts comprising *Tenacity* and unchecked in today's society have created a myriad of problems. These three instincts will be described in detail in the next chapter as the *unholy trinity*. Though adaptive in our past evolutionary history, today they are responsible for many of the world's problems. They rear their ugliness in ways in which we are all too familiar—especially when one group of people are being treated unfairly by another group simply because they are different from the dominant group. Measured Fairness and Compassionate Empathy are certainly challenged in the presence of powerful negative "isms" such as racism, sexism, ageism, and intellectualism. As much as we have witnessed significant increases in antiracism practices over the past one hundred years, many would assert that racist attitudes and practices persist in a strong manner throughout the world. This has led some to wonder when, if ever, racism and all the "isms" for that matter will be erased.

If the natural disposition in each child is to display Measured Fairness, Compassionate Empathy, and the five additional instincts comprising *Tenacity*, one may ask what are the consequences when existing biases and discriminatory practices impede and thwart the normal development of these instincts in many individuals and societies. For those who have experienced racism throughout their lives—racism also faced by their ancestors—it is little wonder that intense feelings of frustration and anger emerge, fueled further by the belief that things will not improve in any appreciable manner. As the late James Baldwin noted in his 1963 book, *The Fire Next Time,* "The most dangerous creation of any society is the man who has nothing to lose."

Another question we might ask is what transpires in the minds of children who grow up in homes in which the practice of racism (or other "isms") is subtly or directly expressed on a regular basis? What parts of their humanity are lost when natural instincts related to caring, compassion, and fairness do not have an opportunity to develop? Similar to those who are oppressed, these children also are filled with anger, resenting and acting out against those whom they perceive as threatening because they are different in some manner. Turning once more to the words of Mr. Baldwin in *The Fire Next Time:* "Please try to remember that what they believe, as well as what they do and cause you to endure, does not testify to your inferiority but to their inhumanity" and "Hatred, which could destroy so much, never failed to destroy the man who hated."

Parents Nurturing Measured Fairness

We have stressed in earlier chapters that as parents strive to reinforce the development of any instinct, they should reflect upon the ways in which they model this instinct and reinforce it in their children. The same is true for the instinct of Measured Fairness. There are ample opportunities during any day or week to accomplish this teaching. How parents relate to each other and to others and how they demonstrate dignity and fairness, play a large role in the development of a child's sense of what is fair and what is not, what is right and what is wrong.

Current events, of which children are more aware of than we may realize, often include incidents of bias and bigotry. It is important for parents to discuss in ways appropriate for the developmental level of their children these events from the perspective of fairness. Parents can also include consideration of other instincts such as Compassionate Empathy and Genuine Altruism as part of this dialogue.

Playing board and card games are another avenue through which parents can model, teach, and practice fairness behaviors such as learning to take turns, playing according to the rules, losing without resentment, and winning without gloating. Parents do not have to give an extended lecture about the importance of fairness, but just naturally build this theme into the game.

If parents do not engage in these kinds of activities or even worse, if they convey actions and messages opposed to fairness, it can be very difficult for children to practice Measured Fairness. This was certainly true for Saul, an 11 year old who frequently resorted to cheating on tests or games and always insisted on going first in any activity. The school counselor strongly recommended to Saul's parents, Stan and Teresa Stiles, that they contact us since she was concerned that Saul's behavior was harming his relationships with peers who as she observed "did not want to play with someone who cheats and who brags about how he is the best at everything." The counselor added that Saul seemed to feel that it's unfair if he doesn't win all of the time and he typically accused others of cheating if he lost. Some anxious children complain of a lack of fairness in games as a consequence of their fear of perceived failure; with Saul, any fear was related to his father.

The counselor also informed us that Stan at first did not want to accept a referral to consult with us, asserting that his son's problems were due in large part because his teachers were not doing a very competent job. She said that Stan was a very competitive man who often dictated his philosophy to his son, which was, "Winning is the only thing. If you don't win, you're a loser." She noted that Teresa rarely said anything at the school meetings and deferred to her husband, who could be very challenging and confrontive with the school staff.

In our individual work with Saul and in our meetings with his parents, it became apparent very quickly that conditional rather than unconditional love and acceptance permeated their home. Saul was painfully aware that his father's acceptance was rooted in his being number one in all of his activities and achieving very high grades in school. Stan's philosophy of success placed a heavy burden on Saul. Any semblance of fairness toward peers or others was sacrificed in his desperation to garner his father's love. It required a considerable amount of intervention on our part, especially with Stan, to alter the script that existed in their house—a script that vividly illustrated the ways in which achievement of Measured Fairness could be derailed by opposing parental values.

The Challenge to Think and Be Fair

Author, Mr. H. Jackson Brown Jr. wrote "Live so that when your children think of fairness and integrity, they think of you." As we've seen, Measured Fairness is represented in various ways. Many research studies have examined equitable sharing, both advantageous and disadvantageous, at different ages and in different countries. On a societal level, a lack of fairness and empathy has for centuries fueled the flames of racism and other "isms" that weaken the fabric of that society. In our clinical practice, we have witnessed and participated in many debates of fairness, frequently represented by questions of "Why me?" or "Why my child?"—questions that are understandable and expected. However, if these questions dominate one's mindset for too long, they deter people from finding solutions and/or purpose to overcome the situation that they perceive as unfair. And we have seen time and time again, misplaced values of success can blind parents from nurturing Measured Fairness in their children.

The reinforcement of the seven instincts comprising *Tenacity* in each child's development is a major responsibility for parents and other caregivers. In order to meet that responsibility successfully, we must not only understand the components of each of the seven instincts but also the negative forces that work against the blossoming of these instincts. This understanding of what we referred to earlier as the *unholy trinity* will provide us with the knowledge to help counter these destructive instincts so that the seven instincts comprising *Tenacity* can thrive. Let us now turn to the *unholy trinity* and our dancing brains.

Chapter 10
Brain Dance

Thirty-five years after we first met and evaluated Andrew, he returned to see us seeking our help. You may recall that Andrew, whom we introduced in Chapter 1, was the young boy with Autism who loved to gaze at the world through the circular opening of a wooden spoon. At six and a half years of age, Andrew decided that his last spoon could be put to better use by someone else. He brought it in a gift-wrapped package telling us he no longer needed it and that we could give it to someone who might need it. When Andrew called and asked for an appointment, he didn't mention the spoon, but we had not forgotten about it and in fact used it often in our talks about Autism.

At forty-one years of age, Andrew was a tall, well-dressed, handsome adult. Meeting us in the waiting room, he quickly made eye contact and offered his hand in a handshake. We walked Andrew back to our office.

"Do you remember me?" Andrew asked. Fortunately our clinic kept very good records. We were able to retrieve Andrew's evaluation and our notes from the electronic database.

"Yes, interestingly enough," we answered. "We have your evaluation and notes right here and your spoon!" We held the spoon up. Without hesitation Andrew said, "That was Agnes, my last spoon." We never knew he had named his spoons.

Andrew gazed away, inconsistently making eye contact as he began to tell us what had transpired over the past thirty-five years in his life. In that period of time, he successfully completed elementary, middle, and high school. He did not socialize very much but had a few close friends with whom he shared interests.

"I came to believe that people would never understand me. Some kids in high school were just plain bullies. It almost seemed like they didn't understand me so they were afraid of me because I was different."

Andrew participated in a proselytizing mission for his church for two years after high school, followed by four years of college and three years of law school. None of this surprised us. Even as a six year old with Autism, Andrew's intelligence was easily observed.

© Springer Nature Switzerland AG 2021
S. Goldstein and R. B. Brooks, *Tenacity in Children*,
https://doi.org/10.1007/978-3-030-65089-6_10

Andrew continued, "After law school, I decided that I should be married. So, I joined a singles group in my church and eventually met and married my wife. We have been married for ten years and have two young children. Though I wasn't very romantic, there must have been something about me that made my wife fall in love with me. Still to this day I have a difficult time understanding her feelings and try as I might, I struggle to explain my thoughts and emotions to her. I try to be a good father to my children, but truth be told, I don't really understand how children think."

We smiled and said nothing. Andrew awkwardly smiled back and continued, "But that's not why I'm here. You see, I'm in my third legal position. All three of my employers were and are impressed with the quality of my work, however all three eventually expressed their concerns that I didn't know how to communicate effectively with clients. They were right. The first two asked me to resign as I would not be promoted to an Associate. I've just been asked to shift my position with my third law firm. Fortunately, the firm I currently work for is large enough that they have offered me a position to analyze and review contracts for a number of very important clients. This position will not require that I communicate with clients nor very many of my colleagues. In fact, they told me that most days I can work from home."

Andrew looked quite sad as he made this comment. He added, "In many ways I am relieved that I can work from home and continue my law career, but I fear that if I don't develop better people skills I'll never advance. Do you think it can ever happen?"

We responded affirmatively and described the very recent research studying camouflage/coping strategies adults with Autism often develop independently through trial and error. We provided Andrew with a number of articles about the types of coping behaviors and strategies that others had found successful and referred him to a community provider, specializing in working with adults with high functioning Autism.

We wondered how much of Andrew's challenges were a consequence of his Autism-related social learning impairments versus the inability of others to accept and embrace differences in others. Or, for that matter convey empathy rather than display aggression toward others who do not fit their comfort level or beliefs. In a 2014 study, the British charity Scope reported that 67% of people feel uncomfortable when talking to a person with any type of disability. Though many mental health experts contend this awkwardness stems from ignorance and fear, evolutionary scientists have offered very different theories about a number of instincts in addition to the seven that we have identified as components of *Tenacity*. Three of these instincts work in an opposite direction in modern society from the seven, creating risk and vulnerability. We call these three—rigid adherence to belief, fear of difference, and defensive aggression—the *unholy trinity*. In combination, they lead us to *brain dance* in times of stress.

Brain Dance

Neuro-anthropologist Dr. Dean Faulk coined the term *brain dance* in her 1992 book of the same title. In defining this term, Dr. Faulk pointed out that despite the popular myth that humans are a calm, considerate, and peaceful species, we are in fact just the opposite. We are all *brain dancing*. At any given minute, our response to any perceived threat or stress in our environment can lead us to lose control of our behavior and act in aggressive and unthinking ways. Dr. Faulk proposed that the evolution of the human brain, from the oldest parts in the back to the more recently evolving front meant that our frontal lobes are not always in control of our actions. It is our frontal lobes that guide us to think rationally and logically in the presence of problems and stress. However, the middle of the brain receives information about the world a few milliseconds before the front of the brain. The middle of the brain guides our response to the world on an emotional basis. As Dr. Faulk points out, the process of maturation involves learning how to provide the front of the brain sufficient time to process what the middle of the brain is already aware of and wanting to act upon. Rather than *brain dance* in the presence of a perceived threat or stress, we can learn to open a window between experience and response, choosing a rational, as opposed to an emotionally driven, solution to problems that confront us.

Unfortunately, we are all prone to *brain dance*. Even the most patient, calm, and rational among us, in the presence of perceived or actual threat or stressful circumstances, can quickly lose control, acting on emotionally driven impulse rather than careful or thoughtful assessment of a problem. Why do we *brain dance*? We believe that the three simple instincts, described earlier, in particular, are responsible for this process. Primitive in their development in our evolutionary history, they were critically important to our survival. We call these *the unholy trinity* because if left unchecked they lead us to chaos. These instincts helped keep us alive for thousands of years, but in recent history are the root of much that ails our species. Andrew in part alluded to these three as he discussed his challenges with peers during his childhood.

The Unholy Trinity

Open a newspaper, visit a web page, or turn to the evening news on your favorite channel. You will find dozens of stories of adverse events in the world on any given day. We maintain these three basic instincts—rigid adherence to belief, fear of difference, and defensive aggression—alone or in combination explain why these events are occurring. Ideological differences are at the root of conflicts between political parties, countries, ethnic groups, religions, or those of different economic classes. The destructive, illegal, and at times unprovoked aggressive actions of many are justified by belief. Each group believes they are right and others wrong. Each group fears the actions of the others. In extreme situations, some groups resort to violence, seeking to have their ideology prevail. It is imperative as a society that we understand that these three basic instincts that once ensured our survival have contributed to destructive events for many centuries. We will define and elaborate each to help you better appreciate our position.

Rigid adherence to belief. Investment advisor and author, Mr. Michael Yardney wrote, "The Law of Belief says that you do not necessarily believe what you see, but you see what you have already decided to believe." Thus, belief can be a valuable ally in the absence of fact. Unfortunately, in present times many of us rigidly adhere to erroneous beliefs even when available facts argue otherwise. For hundreds of thousands of years, our ancestors developed a tenuous relationship with the surrounding environment. How did they know the sun would come up the next day; the weather might turn warm after freezing cold, or, for that matter, if sustenance and shelter would be discovered? The answer is belief. By developing belief, we were able to negotiate an unknown, often dangerous and complex environment. However, absent the application of Simultaneous Intelligence and Measured Fairness, our beliefs are blindly followed sometimes to disaster.

Anthropologist Dr. Augustin Fuentes wrote that "science and rules cannot ensure lasting change without belief—the most creative and destructive ability humans have ever evolved." In his 2019 book *Why We Believe,* Dr. Fuentes explored how many human species, but in particular, we Homo sapiens, evolved this uniquely human capacity over a two million year journey to complex religions, political philosophies, and technologies essentially following a three-step path: from (1) imagination to (2) meaning-making to (3) belief systems. Structural changes in our ancestor's brains helped them generate more effective and expansive mental representations. What emerged was a distinctively human imagination, a capacity that allows us to create and shape our futures, and that also gave rise to the next step in the evolution of belief: meaning-making.

Anthropologists don't know when exactly it happened, but within the last hundred thousand years, humans developed the imagination, the thirst for meaning, and the communication skills necessary for creating explanations of mysterious phenomena. The rise of imagination, Dr. Fuentes argued, sparked positive feedback loops in our brains between creativity, social collaboration, teaching, learning, and experimenting. By at least 40,000 to 50,000 years ago, representational art arose: depictions of hunts, animal–human hybrids, blazing sunsets, and hand prints waving, as if they are signaling. Once groups are attributing shared meaning to objects they can manipulate, it is an easy jump to give shared meaning to larger elements they cannot change: storms, floods, earthquakes, volcanoes, eclipses, and even death.

Through language, deeply held thoughts and ideas could be transferred rapidly and effectively from individuals to small groups to wider populations. This created large-scale shared structures of meaning—what we now call belief systems. Between 4,000 and 15,000 years ago, numerous radical transitions occurred in many human populations. Humans domesticated plants and animals. They developed, along with agriculture, substantial food storage capacities and technologies. Concepts of property and inequality emerged. Towns and, eventually, cities grew. All of this led to the formation of multi-community settlements with stratified political and economic structures. Belief then has served an essential role in our evolutionary history. When applied with respect and care, belief is essential to our future. But when directed to control or harm others or even directed toward ourselves, actions based on misguided belief become a powerful, destructive agent.

In our clinical practice, we have on many occasions witnessed the ways in which negative beliefs become expressed in self-defeating behaviors. We view as a major therapeutic goal, the transformation of negative beliefs into positive beliefs and behaviors. An example of the devastation that a negative belief system can cause on the development of a child or adolescent appeared in our work with David, a 15 year old who was burdened with a number of issues when his father Sy Everett contacted us. David had two older sisters, one who had recently graduated from college and the other who was a sophomore in college. Their mother was diagnosed with an aggressive form of cancer when David was nine years old, and she died a year later.

Sy told us, "David has always struggled in school. He was diagnosed with dyslexia when he was about eight and my wife really helped to make certain he received services at school to help him with his reading. But even with help, it was obvious that David lacked confidence in his ability to learn. The one thing that seemed to bring him any pleasure was that he was an excellent athlete and played several different sports. After my wife died, I tried to do the best I could to make certain that David got extra help and I must say that the school was very supportive. But especially when he started high school last year, you could see a downturn in his behavior. He seemed really discouraged. Not only that, he gave up sports, told me that school 'sucked,' and his grades were really slipping. I was at work and the girls were at college so David came home to an empty house each day and it was difficult to monitor what he was doing."

Sy paused and teared up. "It's been so hard on all of us since my wife died. She held the family together. I feel things are getting worse with David. He used to talk with his sisters, but he rarely does that anymore. I know his mother's death hit him very hard. It's obvious he's depressed and has been for a while. The school recommended I contact a therapist a few years ago, but David was adamant that he was fine and didn't want to see a 'shrink.' I probably should have pushed things, but I didn't want to get into a battle with him. I told him this time he had no choice. As you know, he didn't want to come in today, but said he would come in after I met you."

David came in for his first appointment the following week. There were many dimensions of our intervention during the following year, including sessions with David, meetings with Sy, and eventually with David and Sy, as well as our consultation with his teachers and a tutor. The consultation with his teachers and school counselor led to the Junior Varsity basketball coach reaching out to David to invite him to play the sport he loved the most. We want to highlight at this point one very poignant, dramatic session we had with David that illustrated the pernicious impact of a long-held belief on a youngster's development.

This particular session occurred three months after we began to see David. He looked even more sad than usual when he arrived. We commented on his appearance and without saying anything, he took out a sheet of paper from his backpack. It was a math test that he had failed, one that he told us he thought he would pass. He said, "I've never mentioned this to anyone before, but I think I was born with half a brain."

With a look of desperation on his face, he added, "Is there a way to fill in the other half?" We were startled by what he said.

We knew that it was not easy for David to share this belief, one that we discovered he had been carrying with him for nearly seven years. In hearing what he said, we told him how difficult it must be for him to believe he only had half a brain. We added that we were glad he could tell us. He explained that when he was eight years old he failed a spelling test and a classmate said, "How could you fail a spelling test? You must have half a brain."

David continued, "I knew half of my brain wasn't actually missing, that it was there but that it wasn't working. I thought if someone has half a brain that isn't working, you could only learn half as much as other kids whose entire brains were working."

A simple comment made by a peer to a vulnerable child had a devastating effect. He then lost his mother two years later, who by all accounts was his biggest support. He could not rid himself of the image of half a brain, which intensified his sad, pessimistic mood and left him doubting his ability to succeed in any activities. In the weeks that followed his announcement to us about having half a brain, we focused on shifting this irrational belief by discussing the different strengths and vulnerabilities we all possess. We even talked about the workings of the brain, and, very importantly, emphasized that kids with reading problems could be helped and learn to read.

Years later when we described our work with David at a conference, a man in his mid-50s came up afterward and said he was very moved by the information we shared. He added that until he was diagnosed with reading disabilities five years ago at the age of 50, he had thoughts similar to those held by David. With obvious emotion, he reported, "All my life I thought I was dumb, that my brain was defective, and that I could never get better. There were so many tears shed and years lost until a friend who also has reading problems suggested I get tested. I actually found out I had dyslexia, but I was pretty smart in many areas. Fortunately, David learned much earlier in his life that there was hope. I'm trying not to look at the years I lost but rather the years I still have ahead of me."

Fear of difference. This is the second of the *unholy trinity*. We are afraid of anything different, whether it is the color of someone's skin, their political ideology, or even certain foods. The survival of our ancestors was due, in part, because they avoided difference. Most likely they would forage in the same place, drink from the same water source, and when possible, sleep in places that they had found to be safe and protected. We associated only with those whom we knew, the members of our small family band or tribe. To do otherwise might lead to death. Over thousands of generations, the fear of difference kept us alive but also generalized into our genes and biology.

Eric was a five-year-old child we worked with many years ago. Eric had suffered a near fatal brain injury as a two-year-old child in an automobile accident involving his entire family. Fortunately, no one died, but Eric was the most severely injured. Despite his injuries, over the following two years Eric made an amazing recovery. His development had been advanced prior to the accident. With the support of his family and many caring professionals, his intellect returned and his development continued.

In fact, by four and half years of age he was a near fluent reader. But Eric was not left unscathed. He developed a pattern of restless, often impulsive, rigid behavior leading to emotional outbursts when he became frustrated. As he transitioned into kindergarten, this pattern was reducing but still occurring.

Eric's mother called mid-week with a crisis and asked if she could bring Eric to see us. We had developed a close friendship with Eric over three years. He enjoyed our twice monthly visits. Eric's mother explained that a guest had come into Eric's classroom. His teacher, aware that he was the best reader in the class, asked Eric to read aloud, something he had done before, just not when a visitor was present.

Eric responded to the request with, "You know I can't read, why did you ask me?"

His teacher replied, "But Eric you are our best reader."

Eric resisted again and when gently encouraged by his teacher had an emotional meltdown that escalated until his mother was called to come and take him home. By the time she brought Eric to see us later that afternoon he had returned to his usual happy demeanor.

We asked Eric what happened. Without hesitation he responded, "The teacher asked me to read and I didn't want to so I told her I couldn't read."

"But aren't you a good reader?"

"Yes, I'm the best reader in my class," Eric responded.

Before we could ask another question, Eric continued, "It's not good to be different. If you are different, kids don't like you. I don't want to be different so I told her I can't read, just like my friends."

This led to an interesting discussion with Eric of good or valuable differences versus negative or problematic differences. However, at Eric's age, his thinking was still very black and white. We're not sure he believed us. He promised to apologize to his teacher and ask her in the future that if she wanted him to do something special in class that she ask him privately first. Though Eric wasn't necessarily afraid of difference, he recognized that in order to fit in, he shouldn't be different.

Defensive aggression. We describe the third instinct of the *unholy trinity* as defensive aggression. Defensive aggression is the act of striking out at a perceived or actual threat. Evolutionary explanations of this type of aggression suggest that it serves an important function in terms of both individual survival as well as reproductive potential. Competition arises when resources are limited, and animals must compete in order to survive and reproduce. It is thought that aggressive behavior evolved in males as a method of fighting among themselves. The strongest took the females. We still observe this today in many species. Thus, the development of aggression was similar in males to the development of fancy colors, feathers, and mating dances, all designed to attract females. Unfortunately, evolutionary history reflects that males did not simply abandon their aggressive nature as all members of the deer family do with large racks of antlers once mating season ends and females are impregnated. Instead they turned their aggression against females as a means of control. Aggression is a characteristic trait of both genders of our species, more so a problem among men. In times of stress as Dr. Faulk points out, we are prone to respond aggressively rather than thoughtfully.

Not everyone agrees with this theory of aggression, however. Some argue that aggression is not instinctual but learned behavior in response to environmental threat and that evolution has wired us to be peaceful and composed. Though it may seem easier to divide the debate into two camps—those who think evolution has made humans naturally peaceful and those who think we're more naturally prone to violence, the real answer probably lies somewhere in between, according to Dr. Elizabeth Cashdan, a professor of anthropology at the University of Utah. At a 2019 conference on violence and human evolution, Dr. Cashdan argued, "There is plenty of evidence to support both claims: violence, reconciliation, and cooperation are all part of human nature." She believes these wide-ranging emotions evolved because they benefited humans in some way in the past. Evolution, Dr. Cashden pointed out, can explain why we are prone to pro or reactive aggression. In her view, it is a primal emotion like any other.

During the process of evaluating countless young children with language delays over the course of our careers, we have observed patterns of aggressive behavior displayed when language was unavailable to these children. These children often struggled to shift from a tactile way of processing their world to one guided by language. Young children with language delay must touch and feel everything in the environment because they lack the vocabulary to classify objects. We have observed in many such children that as they acquire functional language their patterns of unprovoked or reactionary aggression are replaced with words directed at others. Three-year-old Lynsey was Paul and Linda Coen's only child. She was a very normal appearing child. However, at 3 years of age, Lynsey was barely speaking. Her parents enrolled her in preschool hoping the socialization experience would stimulate her language development. Lynsey's pediatrician was concerned she may have Autism. We met with them one morning for a consultation while Lynsey was at preschool.

We began by asking the Coen's what they liked about Lynsey. Without hesitation they jointly answered, "Her loving personality."

We asked them to elaborate. Paul continued, "Lynsey loves to snuggle and give hugs. We can take her almost anywhere and she is well behaved, but like any child she struggles with her emotions when tired. Lynsey's big problem is her lack of speech. She seems to understand very well but still speaks in single words. Being first time parents, we didn't think this was a big problem till we enrolled her in preschool. She did fine the first day until she had a disagreement with another child and then she bit him! We don't really think Lynsey is Autistic, but we want to make sure we're doing all we can to help her."

"We tried to discipline her with time out," added Linda, "but after biting a third child in her first week of preschool she was asked to leave. I never thought our child would be expelled from preschool. We've enrolled her in another preschool, but she is already having problems."

After taking a full history and evaluating a number of behavioral questionnaires the Coen's had completed, it was clear that Lynsey's delay in spoken language was just that and not an early emerging sign of broad developmental delay such as Autism or emotional problems. We explained this to the Coens and referred them to a community-based speech language pathologist. Further, we helped the Coens understand that just as you wouldn't place a beginner swimmer in a class to learn the butterfly stroke, a regular preschool at this time was not a good fit for Lynsey. We also referred the Coens to a preschool designed for children with language delays. This was a better fit for Lynsey.

We had the opportunity to evaluate Lynsey two years later before she entered kindergarten. Her speech had blossomed and along with it so too had her social skills. She no longer resorted to biting or any aggressive act for that matter when upset but could now "use her words."

The Solution Before Us

Fifty thousand years ago acting on these three basic instincts under stress that reflected real or perceived threat, increased our chances of survival. Today we would argue that when left unchecked these three—rigid adherence to belief, fear of difference, and defensive aggression—are responsible for much we see wrong with our world and society today.

Author and zoologist Dr. Clive Bromhall points out in his classic 2004 book, *The Eternal Child*, that in our evolutionary development we sacrificed all means of protection from the environment around us. We shifted to walking on two legs when four was more efficient. We gave up thick skin and protective hair. We walked with our heads erect, open to the hot sun of the African Savannah. However, in exchange, all of our evolutionary energy was focused on building a bigger, more complex brain. The seven instincts of *Tenacity* developed and evolved because of this brain. The *unholy trinity* of the three instincts we describe in this chapter developed as well for the very same reason, and we believe even earlier than the seven instincts comprising *Tenacity*.

However, our role as parents, caregivers, and educators is just the opposite with these three instincts. Instead of creating experiences for these three instincts to develop and blossom, we work for just the opposite—to help children, everyone for that matter, understand, manage, and thereby minimize the adverse outcomes that will occur when these three are left unchecked or worse, reinforced. By providing children with opportunities to develop the instincts comprising *Tenacity*, we strengthen these instincts and increase children's ability to manage irrational beliefs, be accepting of difference, and solve problems without resorting to aggression.

One Hundred Years in the Future

We always enjoyed our visits with eleven-year-old Nikko. We began working with Nikko almost ten years ago because from a very young age there had been a disconnect between the hypersensitivity of Nikko's nervous system and the world around him. By age two, he was literally afraid of his shadow. By age three, he refused to leave his mother's side. Clowns and circuses scared him. He wouldn't even consider trying the children's rides at the local amusement park or tasting new foods. He resisted entering kindergarten. Every year starting back to school was a challenge. Nikko is very bright but to add to the gauntlet of his childhood he struggled to become an average reader. Nikko was a voracious consumer of science and history programs on television. He enjoyed listening to books on tape. During one visit, Nikko adamantly questioned the wisdom of his teacher's insistence that he learn to read, claiming reading was "old school" and the future of learning lay in television and the Internet.

During one of our most memorable visits with Nikko, he arrived excited to tell us about the new program his dad had loaded into his computer. A program that could read text aloud. Now he was more convinced than ever that he did not need to read. As our discussion about the wonders of computers continued Nikko exclaimed, "You know what? One hundred years from now they will find a way to turn our brains into computers."

"Aren't they like computers now?" we asked.

"Oh no" he answered. "Someday they will just program our brains while we sleep and everyone will read well. Not only that, no one will ever worry because computers aren't people, they're not afraid."

We could almost see the wheels turning in Nikko's mind so we waited. Then a somewhat sad look appeared on Nikko's face. "I guess that wouldn't be so good because then we would never be happy. You can't program a computer to be happy, it's just something you feel."

Computer chips and hard drives are "born" on the assembly line as tabula rasa. Tabula rasa (clean slate in Latin) is the theory that individuals are born without built-in mental content and therefore all knowledge comes from experience or perception. It is a theory that applies much better to computers than people. The genetics of our species make us appear as homunculus (Latin for a small human), like a rose unfolding. While it is true that our brains begin life with a set of reflexes we were never taught, many years ago it was incorrectly thought that all we were and would become was determined by the programming of our genes. But as we've written in this book, biology is not destiny. Growth and development through childhood are a complex dance between nature and nurture. The unfolding of that rose, its health and ultimate beauty, is critically dependent on the world around it. Leave a dozen roses in your hot car for too long, and they will never blossom. The computer may be faster at doing logical things like computations. However, the brain is far better at interpreting the outside world and creating new ideas. In his 2020 book *The Idea of the Brain*, Dr. Matthew Cobb, a professor of biological sciences, addressed this conundrum writing: "Despite the latest buzzwords that zip about—blockchain, quantum supremacy (or quantum anything), nanotech, and so on—it is unlikely that these fields will transform either technology or our view of what brains do."

We Are Self Aware

No matter how advanced our programming algorithms evolve to guide a computer's decision-making or ability to acquire knowledge, we will never program instinct. Nor for that matter will we create software to replace empathy, responsibility, fairness, altruism, optimism, or motivation. We may teach a computer to analyze data simultaneously but it will operate only within the parameters we assign. Computers possess no consciousness nor awareness of their existence. Dr. Michael Graziano, a professor of psychology and neuroscience at Princeton University, wrote in his 2018 book *The Spaces Between Us: A Story of Neuroscience, Evolution, and Human Nature*, that consciousness arose as a solution to one of the most fundamental problems facing any nervous system: too much information from the environment constantly flowing in through our senses to be processed. The brain evolved increasingly sophisticated mechanisms for deeply processing a few select signals at the expense of others. He suggests, consciousness is the ultimate result of that evolutionary sequence. Consciousness he expresses "is an ability that evolved gradually over the past half billion years and is present in a range of vertebrate species."

From our perspective, consciousness and self-awareness are not the same. Consciousness is most likely reflected in the sequence of increasing cognitive complexity children progress through in their thinking as they advance through childhood. It is a series of stages reflecting certain ways of thinking and processing their experiences. We view self-awareness as a discrete phenomenon. It is or it isn't something an organism can do. It is the ability to gaze into a mirror and recognize the person you see as you and be aware that you exist. Very few species besides humans possess this capacity. Research demonstrates great apes, elephants, and dolphins are but a few. Dr. Graziano may be correct that consciousness evolved in small steps, but we wonder how evolution can truly explain the development of self-awareness in a slow, piecemeal fashion. Self-awareness is not like an eye or ear evolving over millions of years in small adaptive steps. You are either aware of your existence or not. Some may even argue that our self-awareness is perhaps the best reason to believe in a divine creator.

The world has changed more in the last 45 years since we started our work as psychologists than in the previous one hundred years or more. Accompanying these rapid advances have been equally developing adversities, many of our own making. The evolution of technology races ahead at breakneck speeds. We worry that this frenetic speed is quickly outpacing our human capacity to cope and adapt, to harness and effectively utilize our instincts not just to survive but to thrive. British novelist, Ms. Zadie Smith wrote: "The past is always tense, the future perfect." Activist Mahatma Ghandi, best known for his non-violent methods of protest, advised: "The future depends on what you do today."

We are cautiously optimistic that as our understanding of ourselves and our place in the Universe grows, we will find the means to better understand our instincts and prepare the next generations to lead us into a promising, though not likely, perfect future. The strength of our conviction is drawn not just from the knowledge we have conveyed in this book, but from the thousands of children and families from whom we have learned time and time again about the tenacity, resiliency, self-discipline, and creativity of the human mind and spirit.

References

Abrami, P., Bernard, R. M., Borokhovski, E., & Wade, A. (2008). Instructional interventions affecting critical thinking skills and dispositions: A stage 1 meta-analysis. *Review of Educational Research, 78*(4), 1102–1134.

Allworth, J. (2012). Empathy: The most valuable thing they teach at HBS. *Harvard Business Review.* https://hbr.org/2012/05/empathy-the-most-valuable-thing

American Association for the Advancement of Science. (2015). Kids' altruism linked with better physiological regulation less family wealth. *EurekaAlert!* https://www.eurekalert.org/pub_rel eases/2015-06/afps-kal060115.php

Baldwin, J. (1963). *The fire next time.* New York: Random House.

Baumeister, R., & Leary, M. R. (1995). The need to belong: Desire for interpersonal attachments as a fundamental human motivation. *Psychological Bulletin, 117*(3), 497–529.

Blake, P. R. (2015). It's not fair! *Boston University Newsletter.* https://www.bu.edu/articles/2015/child-development-fairness

Blake, P. R., McAuliffe, K., Corbit, J., Callaghan, T. C., Barry, O., Bowie, A., et al. (2015). The ontogeny of fairness in seven societies. *Nature, 528,* 258–262.

Bromhall, C. (2004). *The eternal child: How evolution has made children of us all.* London: Ebury Press.

Brooks, R., & Goldstein, S. (2001). *Raising resilient children.* New York: McGraw-Hill.

Brooks, R., & Goldstein, S. (2002). *Nurturing resilience in our children.* New York: McGraw-Hill.

Brooks, R., & Goldstein, S. (2009). *Raising a self-disciplined child.* New York: McGraw-Hill.

Brooks, R., & Goldstein, S. (2012). *Raising resilient children with autism spectrum disorders.* New York: McGraw-Hill.

Brosnan, S. (2006). Nonhuman species' reactions to inequity and their implications for fairness. *Social Justice Research, 19*(2), 153–185. https://sarah-brosnan.com

Cashdan, E. (2019). Human behavior & evolution society. https://meetatbu.com/hbes19/files/2019/05/HBES-2019-Program-webFinal.pdf

Charity Scope Study. (2014). https://www.scope.org.uk/media/press-releases/brits-feel-uncomfort able-with-disabled-people

Cobb, M. (2020). *The idea of the brain: The past and future of neuroscience.* New York: Basic Books.

Csikszentmihalyi, M. (1990). *Flow: The psychology of optimal experience.* New York: Harper-Collins.

Cyr, D. (2003). An interview with Christopher reeve. *US Airways Attaché Magazine.*

Davidson, R. (2016). The four keys to well-being. *Greater Good Magazine.* https://greatergood.ber keley.edu/article/item/the_four_keys_to_well_being

Deci, E., & Flaste, R. (1996). *Why we do what we do: Understanding self-motivation.* London: Penguin Books.

© Springer Nature Switzerland AG 2021
S. Goldstein and R. B. Brooks, *Tenacity in Children,*
https://doi.org/10.1007/978-3-030-65089-6

Deci, E. L., & Ryan, R. M. (1985). *Intrinsic motivation and self-determination in human behavior.* New York: Plenum Publishing Company.

deWaal, F. (2005). The evolution of empathy. *Greater Good Magazine.* https://greatergood.berkeley.edu/article/item/the_evolution_of_empathy

deWaal, F. B. M., & Brosnan, S. (2014) Evolution of responses to (un)fairness. *Science, 346* (6207) Washington DC: American Association for the Advancement of Science.

Dewar, G. (2009–2012) Teaching critical thinking: An evidence-based guide. https://www.parentingscience.com/teaching-critical-thinking.html

Ekman, P. (2010). Taxonomy of compassion. *Greater Good Magazine.* https://greatergood.berkeley.edu/article/item/paul_ekmans_taxonomy_of_compassion

Faulk, D. (1992). *Brain dance.* New York: Henry Holt and Company.

Fehr, E., & Schmidt, K. (1999) A theory of fairness, competition, and cooperation. *The Quarterly Journal of Economics, 114*(3). Oxford: Oxford University Press.

Fuentes, A. (2019). *Why we believe: Evolution and the human way of being.* London: Yale University Press.

Geirland, J. (1996). Go with the flow. https://www.wired.com/1996/09/czik

Goldman, B. (2017). The power of kindness: Why empathy is essential in our everyday lives. *Roots of Empathy Research Symposium, Toronto.* https://rootsofempathy.org/wp-content/uploads/2017/11/2016-Symposium-Proceedings.pdf

Goldstein, S., & Brooks, B. (Eds.). (2005). *Handbook of resilience in children.* New York: Springer.

Goldstein, S., & Brooks, B. (Eds.). (2013). *Handbook of resilience in children* (2nd ed.). New York: Springer.

Goleman, D., Boyatzis, R., & McKee, A. (2002). *Primal leadership: Realizing the power of emotional intelligence.* Boston: Harvard Business School Press.

Gorlick, A. (2008). For kids, altruism comes naturally. *Stanford News.* https://news.stanford.edu/news/2008/november5/tanner-110508.html

Graziano, M. (2018). *The spaces between us: A story of neuroscience, evolution, and human nature.* New York: Oxford University Press.

Grover, S. (2015). Four ways altruism produces happy and empowered children. *Psychology Today.* https://www.psychologytoday.com/intl/blog/when-kids-call-the-shots/201511/4-ways-altruism-produces-happy-and-empowered-children

Harvard Health Publishing. (2008). Optimism and your health. Harvard Health Publishing. https://www.health.harvard.edu/heart-health/optimism-and-your-health

Herrnstein, R. J., Nickerson, R. S., Sanchez, M., & Swets, J. A. (1986). Teaching thinking skills. *American Psychologist, 41,* 1279–1289.

Keltner, D. (2012). What is compassion? *Greater Good Magazine.* https://greatergood.berkeley.edu/topic/compassion/definition

Kohn, A. (1993). *Punished by rewards.* Boston: Houghton Mifflin Harcourt.

Konnikova, M. (2016). How we learn fairness. *New Yorker Magazine.* https://www.newyorker.com/science/maria-konnikova/how-we-learn-fairness

Lavoie, R. (2007). *The motivation breakthrough.* New York: Atria Press

Lee, L. O., James, P., Zevon, E. S., Kim, E. S., Trudel-Fitzgerald, C., Spiro III, A., Grodstein, F., & Kubzansky. (2019). Optimism is associated with exceptional longevity in 2 epidemiologic cohorts of men and women. *Proceedings of the American Academy of Sciences of the USA.* https://www.pnas.org/content/116/37/18357

Lepper, M. R., Greene, D., & Nisbett, R. E. (1973). Undermining children's intrinsic interest with extrinsic reward: A test of the "overjustification" hypothesis. *Journal of Personality and Social Psychology, 28,* 129–137.

Li, J., Wang, W., Jing, Y., & Zhu, L. (2016). Young children's development of fairness. *Frontiers of Psychology.* https://doi.org/10.3389/fpsyg.2016.01274.

Luria, A. R. (1976). *The working brain.* London: Penguin Books.

Marsh, J. (2012). The power of self-compassion: An interview with Kristin Neff. *Greater Good Magazine.* https://greatergood.berkeley.edu/article/item/the_power_of_self_compassion

Meltzoff, A. (2017). Research on attachment relationship. *Roots of Empathy Research Symposium, Toronto.* https://rootsofempathy.org/wp-content/uploads/2017/11/2016-Symposium-Proceedings.pdf

Mercier, H., & Sperber, D. (2017). *The enigma of reason.* Cambridge: Harvard University Press.

Moran, B. (2016). "It's not fair!" A study of how children learn to share. *Boston University College of Arts & Sciences Magazine.* https://www.bu.edu/cas/magazine/spring16/its-not-fair

Morris, A., & Frei, F. (2012). *Uncommon service: How to win by putting customers at the core of your business.* Cambridge: Harvard Business Review Press.

Oettingen, G. (2014). *Rethinking positive thinking: Inside the new science of motivation.* New York: Penguin Books.

Palmer, T. (1822). *Teacher's manual: Being an exposition of an efficient and economical system of education suited to the wants of a free people.* London England: Forgotten Books.

Peterson, C. (2000). The future of optimism. *American Psychologist, 55,* 44–55.

Pink, D. H. (2009). *Drive.* New York: Riverhead Books.

Pinker, S. (1994). *The language instinct.* New York: Harper Collins.

Proctor, D., Williamson, R., de Waal, F. B. M., & Brosnan, S. (2013). Chimpanzees play the ultimatum game. *Proceedings of the National Academy of Sciences, 110*(6), 2070–2075. https://doi.org/10.1073/pnas.1220806110.

Ridley, M. (2011). *The rational optimist.* New York: HarperCollins.

Ryan, R. M., & Deci, E. L. (2017). *Self-determination theory: Basic psychological needs in motivation, development, and wellness.* New York: Guilford Press.

Sack, D. (2012). From mine to ours: Nurturing empathy in children. *Huffington Post.* https://www.huffpost.com/entry/empathy_b_1658984

Sandal, M. (2020). Why some Americans refuse to social distance and wear masks. *The Harvard Gazette.* https://news.harvard.edu/gazette/story/2020/08/sandel-explores-ethics-of-what-we-owe-each-other-in-a-pandemic

Schairer, S. (2017). What's the difference between empathy, sympathy, and compassion? Chopra Center. https://chopra.com/articles

Scheier, M. F., & Carver, C. (1992). Effects of optimism on psychological and physical well-being. *Cognitive Therapy and Research, 16,* 201–228.

Schunk, D. H. (1983). Ability versus effort attributional feedback: Differential effects on self-efficacy and achievement. *Journal of Educational Psychology, 75,* 848–856.

Schunk, D. H. (1984). Sequential attributional feedback and children's achievement behaviors. *Journal of Educational Psychology, 76,* 1159–1169.

Schunk, D. H., & Cox, P. D. (1986). Strategy training and attributional feedback with learning disabled students. *Journal of Educational Psychology, 78,* 201–209.

Schunk, D. H., & Zimmerman, B. J. (1997). Social origins of self-regulatory competence. *Educational Psychologist, 32,* 195–208.

Segal, J. (1988). Teachers have enormous power in attracting a child's self-esteem. *Brown University Child Behavior and Development Newsletter, 10,* 1–3.

Seligman, M. E. P. (2006). *Learned optimism: How to change your mind and your life.* New York: Vintage Books.

Shure, M. B. (1996). *Raising a thinking child.* New York: Pocket Books.

Shure, M. B. (2001). *Raising a thinking preteen.* New York: Owl/Holt.

Smith, C. (2016). How children's sense of fairness changes as they age. *Newsletter of the Center for Human Growth & Development*, University of Michigan. https://chgd.umich.edu/how-childrens-sense-of-fairness-changes-as-they-age

Vallerand, R. J., & Reid, G. (1984). On the causal effects of perceived competence on intrinsic motivation: A test of cognitive evaluation theory. *Journal of Sport Psychology, 6,* 94–102.

Walsh, E., & Walsh, D. (2019). How children develop empathy. *Psychology Today.* https://www.psychologytoday.com/intl/blog/smart-parenting-smarter-kids/201905/how-children-develop-empathy

Warneken, F. (2010). On the origins of altruism in ontogeny and phylogeny. *Boston University Dialogues on Biological Anthropology.* https://www.bu.edu/anthrop/files/2010/10/Warneken_sta tement.pdf

Warneken, F., & Tomasello, M. (2006). Altruistic helping in human infants and young Chimpanzees. *Science, 311,* 1301–1303.

Warneken, F., & Tomasello, M. (2009). The roots of human altruism. *British Journal of Psychology, 100,* 455–471.

Weiner, B. (1974). *Achievement motivation and attribution theory.* Morristown, NJ: General Learning Press.

White, R. (1959). Motivation reconsidered: The concept of competence. *Psychological Review, 66,* 297–333.

Zohar, A., Weinberger, Y., & Tamir, P. (1994). The effect of the biology critical thinking project on the development of critical thinking. *Journal of Research in Science Teaching, 31*(2), 183–196.

Author Index

© Springer Nature Switzerland AG 2021
S. Goldstein and R. B. Brooks, *Tenacity in Children*,
https://doi.org/10.1007/978-3-030-65089-6

Subject Index

© Springer Nature Switzerland AG 2021
S. Goldstein and R. B. Brooks, *Tenacity in Children*,
https://doi.org/10.1007/978-3-030-65089-6